Halfway
A Journal through Pregnancy

Katherine Cottle

Halfway
A Journal through Pregnancy

Katherine Cottle

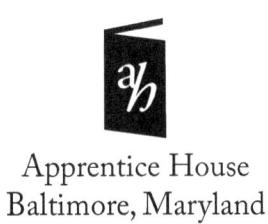

Apprentice House
Baltimore, Maryland

ALSO BY KATHERINE COTTLE

Poetry
My Father's Speech (2008)

"A pregnancy diary, one would think, has a predictable ending. Not this one. The suspense is all but unbearable throughout *Halfway*. Though movie-like in its artful cuts from story to story, now to then, dream-time to real-time, prose to poetry, it suggests a movie that is perhaps too graphic to be made, one that is as gruellingly unflinching as the title of the book's first section: The Clot Baby. The book is exhausting, horrifying, and deeply gratifying."

    - Clarinda Harriss, Towson University
       Author of *Dirty Blue Voice* & *Air Travel*

"*Halfway* is a captivating depiction of pregnancy as a roller coaster of hopes, anxieties, disappointments, and dreams. Cottle's prose is lyrical, poignant, and exquisitely crafted—it makes you want to keep reading and rereading. A stunning first memoir."

    - Michelle M. Tokarczyk, Goucher College
       Author of *Class Definitions* & *Working Class Women in the Academy*

© 2010 by Katherine Cottle

ISBN: 978-1-934074-50-3

All rights reserved. No part of this book may be reproduced or transmitted in any form or by any means, electronic or mechanical, including photocopy, recording, or any information storage and retrieval system, without prior permission from the publisher (except by reviewers who may quote brief passages).

Printed in the United States of America

First Edition

Published by Apprentice House
The Future of Publishing…Today!

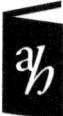

Apprentice House
Communication Department
Loyola University Maryland
4501 N. Charles Street
Baltimore, MD 21210

410.617.5265
410.617.2198 (fax)
www.ApprenticeHouse.com
info@ApprenticeHouse.com

Acknowledgments

I must thank my family for all of their unconditional support and help with writing this memoir. My husband, Jeff Anderson, never let me give up hope. My parents, Harvey and Joyce Cottle, allowed me to believe in myself as a writer since my first kindergarten poem. My siblings, Ben and Abby Cottle, provided the fights and love necessary to keep my writing alive. Joyce Cottle, Shannon Bishop, Shelley Puhak, Carolyn Nair, Michelle Tokarczyk, Stephanie Levin, Alanna McGeary, Amanda Merson, Gregg Wilhelm, Kevin Atticks and Alyssa DeLisio deserve credit for all of the time spent reading my earlier drafts and providing me with constructive feedback. I will never forget the true beginning of this book, which was the inspiration of my former teachers and mentors: Bill Jones, Michelle Tokarczyk, Elizabeth Spires, Madison Smartt Bell, Reginald McKnight and Michael Collier. They taught me to love words and to let the language tell its own story. For that, I am forever grateful.

I would like to give acknowledgment to the following publications for originally printing the included poems and story: "Birdman, Springfield Hospital," *Hungry As We Are* (20th year anniversary edition, editor Ann Darr). Washington D.C. Washington Writers' Publishing House, 1995; "Halfway," *The Best of Artscape 2001 Literary Arts Award Chapbook.* Baltimore, Maryland, 2001; "The beat is within," *Riverwind.* Nelsonville, Ohio, Issue 27, Spring 2004; "First Trimester," *I Will Bear This Scar,* editor Marietta W. Bratton, 2005; "The Miscarriage," *Mourning Sickness: Stories and Poems about Miscarriage, Stillbirth, and Infant Loss*, editors Missy Martin and Jesse Loren, 2008.

To Addison

"Few or no words were spoken and the silent ship, as if manned by painted sailors in wax, day after day tore on through all the swift madness and gladness of the demonic waves."

–*Moby Dick*, Melville

Part One

The Clot Baby

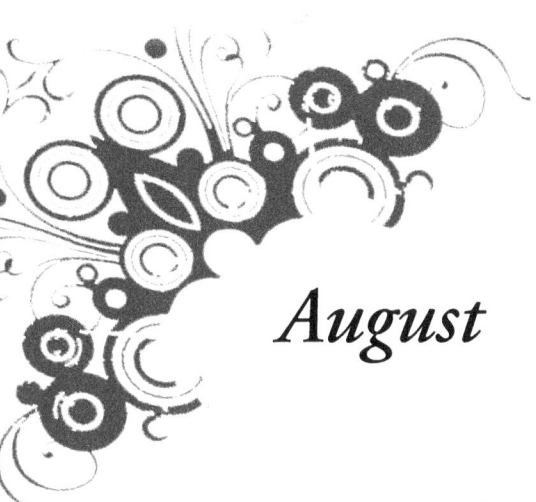

August

"It will be okay. I will take care of you," I whispered to the clot baby, as I draped my ten-year-old arms around its slick torso and rested my chin in the well of its neck. I knew that the rest of the world would not stay by its side, frightened by its body's tangle of soft bone and wet tissue. I was the only one who understood its featureless face, the long sinew in the place of a nose, an empty socket gaping where a mouth should be.

I was a gentle nurse, swabbing the drips from its forehead and wrapping its legs with white towels that were immediately stained bright red with blood. I wanted us to grow up together, to kneel for nighttime prayers beside our twin mattress, zippered up tight inside a thick waterproof plastic cover.

~

That was my reoccurring dream the year after my mother told me about her miscarriage, the pregnancy she had before mine, the one that ended up as a fist of tight clots in the toilet when she was already three months along.

"Could you tell if it was a girl or a boy?" I asked my mother after she described her ordeal.

"No. It was too young, too young to be a real baby," she replied.

"So it was a pretend baby?" I asked, unsure about the whole pregnancy time line and where pretend became real in the equation.

"No, honey, it wasn't pretend, but it wasn't real either. There was something wrong with it, and it wouldn't have ever become a normal baby."

"What was wrong with it?" I wondered.

She paused, thinking about the next step in her explanation.

"I don't know. But I do know that if I had given birth to that baby, I never would have had you."

I remember thinking it wasn't fair, my pushing that baby out of the way without any consideration, so that I could tumble out into the world and land in my mother's arms.

~

That same year our teacher asked us to imagine what we would be doing in two decades. It would be the year of the millennium, and we would have to write the awkward date, 2000, in the top right hand corner of our papers.

"I will be a teacher," I wrote in cursive on the dry yellow paper with the dotted blue lines, "with four cats and twin girls named Lucy and Nancy." I was already on Book #22 of the Nancy Drew Series.

However, I could not imagine I would ever really be that old. That was how old my mother was, with her perm of salt and pepper curls, her calloused feet, and her chicken skin arms. *Thirty* was another life that I could not comprehend, one with checkbooks and ironing boards, and oven temperatures that had their own systematic logic. That life was way down the road. All I could imagine was a pavement that ran past slick skyscrapers and dark forests, and a trolley that would drop me off somewhere in between them.

She did not tell us time would quicken each year as we approached that rounded number. She left out the fact that we were already the same people we would be at thirty, only smaller and without as much grief. She did not let on that aging was like being continually pulled apart at the joints, yet with never enough time or energy to heal.

She smiled as she collected our papers, then read them to herself and cried while we were out at recess, her own list buried in the back of her memory box at home, her predictions of "mother" and "ballerina" still unfulfilled.

~

I filled in the date, *August 2, 2000,* on the new medical history form the nurse had handed to me on the clear plastic clipboard. I wrote 0 on the blank asking for the number of previous pregnancies and noticed a lack of questions about my number of pets or my favorite reading material. *"Are you currently pregnant?"* the next line asked, and I hesitated before checking the *NO* square. There needed to be a follow-up statement that read, *Support your findings in a concise three paragraph essay on the back of this form.* NO did not tell my whole story, and the reason I was sitting there with the unsettling worry I might not even be able to get pregnant. There was no room to write that I was scared I was not qualified to have a child; my house was not big enough, we didn't make enough money, and I always burned the meals. I needed to attach another piece of paper to explain I did not feel like a mother, and I was not sure if that was a prerequisite for pregnancy. *NO* didn't show the number of infertile women in my extended family and the fear of miscarriage that I had carried in my heart like a heavy iron since elementary school.

I finished the form and handed it back, the pen carefully pinched under the metal teeth of the clipboard.

"Come on back, hon," the nurse instructed and motioned me through the door separating the lobby from the examination rooms. She led me into the first room on the left. "Here you go, hon," she continued, handing me what looked like a large paper towel. "Everything off. Put the gown on with the opening in the front. He'll be with you in a minute." After she closed the door, I took off my clothes and piled them according to size on the chair next to the examining table. I wanted to look neat and organized, my responsibility visible in the way I had lined my shoes up directly under the plastic chair with the heels touching.

I heard footsteps slowing down outside the door and the light shuffling of papers. I pulled my paper gown tighter around my middle. The doctor knocked and entered the room.

"Hello. How are you today?"

"We're thinking about trying soon," I blurted out, sure that he could see my plans for fertility already highlighted across my forehead.

"Great," he responded, and pulled two beige rubber gloves out of the box on the sink cabinet.

I had expected him to hand me a *Ten Steps to Proper Pregnancy* list, or to hook me up to the lie detector that had to be hidden behind the locked door at the end of the hall. I had assumed I would have to answer hundreds of questions to determine if I would be a fit parent.

Instead, he instructed me to lie down, to put my feet into the metal stirrups, and to relax while he buzzed the nurse. I tried to relax, to feel like my entire rear end was not hanging off the end of the table and the cold speculum didn't feel like a pair of refrigerated salad tongs. But, like usual, it required an additional *"Relax more!"* before he was able to complete the exam and hand the Pap smear Q-tip over to the nurse in the background. All the while I waited for him to pull out a pregnancy pop quiz from his pocket with a standardized answer sheet ready for my number two pencil.

"Everything looks good. See you in a year, if not before," he winked, as he headed for the door. "You'll only hear back from us if there is a problem with the Pap smear. You can get dressed now."

I was in shock. There were no signed contracts or sworn affidavits, no pledges or badges for my aging Girl Scout sash in my mother's attic. After I was dressed, I wandered back up to the receptionist's desk, feeling like I had lost my wallet or my nighttime bite plate.

The nurse didn't even notice me. For that matter, she barely even registered that I was stamping my parking ticket or taking one of the complimentary, *Pregnancy and You*, magazines that were sitting on the ledge of the window. She was too busy sending out exam reminder postcards with bright gold sunsets and the words *Remember your health!* dancing in unbroken cursive across the bottom.

~

"I think tonight should be the night," I announced to my husband. After all, it was almost the end of the summer, and it is common knowledge that magical events are more likely to occur in the summer, with the last flickers of lightening bugs throughout the backyard and the sticky scent of egg custard snowballs floating up the street. I could see the stars beginning to line up above the house like constellations preparing for a night game. *Hurry*, each figure pleaded with me, before practicing the next curveball towards the chimney.

The damp grass under my bare feet signaled that the hours were ticking by, and it would not be long before the blades started to yellow and shrivel back into the ground. The lawnmower gave me its approval too, completely weary of its seasonal chore. It nodded toward the rusty red gas can resting in the back of the shed like a WWII artifact, a half inch of gasoline still settled in the crusty base.

Maybe it was just the dizziness from the last day at the Maryland State Fair that I was feeling; walking by the leftover Elvis prints and four-feet tall Tweety Birds taped up to the portable walls of the booths, my stomach still burping from the fried dough and cheap beer. Or, maybe it was knowing the carnival would pack up the next day and the Ferris wheel would disappear for another year, along with the crooked steps of the fun house and the carnies, as they stamped out the last of their cigarette butts and closed the doors to their trailers before moving on to the next city.

Most likely it was just the fact that I didn't want another year to go by unnoticed. I didn't want to be the same person back at the fair the next summer, picking up a yellow duck floating in the trash bucket that was supposed to be a duck pond with the fading number three barely visible on its mildewed belly.

"For what?" my husband replied to my announcement.

~

I relaxed in the bathtub, sure that my road to motherhood had just begun. I could almost feel the tiny sperm inside me, doing the butterfly stroke in record time, battling to reach the egg that waited in the far reaches of my uterus like a big raft. It was hard to imagine that there were thousands of them, paddling forward in a life or death struggle. It had to look like a microscopic fleet, headed through rough waters to conquer a new land.

In high school, the sex education films always depicted the sperm with faces, sly grins that showed their eagerness to keep swimming towards the finish line. In one movie the fastest sperm even spoke: "I see it up ahead," he yelled to his fellow comrades like a true captain, then signaled them along with the quick flip of his tail. The entire class laughed, though we girls secretly squirmed in our seats. There was something very sinister about an army of beings ready to invade our bodies at any moment. It was enough to keep all of our legs together, at least for a few months.

That night, I went on pure faith that the competition was still on as I sank my shoulders down into the bubbles and watched the warm water rise up the sides of the tub. I thought I would feel like more of an active participant in the conception process. Instead, I felt like a blind spectator, sitting on the sidelines without my sunglasses. Perhaps, I thought, I should be doing something more to encourage the sperm's success, like standing on my head or holding my breath, instead of just soaking and letting the race continue on its own.

~

Before twenty four hours had passed, I convinced myself that the swimmers had stopped short at the rope separating the shallow end from the deep end of my uterus. I could see them there, afraid to move past the knotted line, their tails huddled in frightened clumps.

The next night I kept my knees propped up on five pillows, just to be safe. I wasn't taking any more chances. I started to believe that one wrong tilt of my hips would cause a detour in their path, or worse yet, create a new current that could withstand any paddle.

"Don't think about it so much," my husband said after he saw me carefully slide another pillow under the stack that was already climbing up towards the ceiling.

"I'm just trying to ensure the most fertile atmosphere," I informed him, ignoring the fact that my feet were starting to go numb.

"Okay," he replied, and I saw his eyes roll as he put the latest issue of *Popular Hotrodding* down on the nightstand. However, I wasn't concerned about his eyes, or the blond woman in a red bikini standing in front of the new Corvette on the cover of the magazine; I was trying to center myself, to keep all energy flowing inward so that nothing could jeopardize this attempt at conception. I laid perfectly still, trying not to scratch the itch on my leg, afraid that one wrong move might destroy all my chances of pregnancy. It felt a lot like a game of hide-and-seek, only this time I was not hiding from my little sister, as I crunched into a fetal ball in the secret compartment under the basement stairs, but from the will of my own body.

~

My knife cut through the chicken breast and made a deep ridge into the cheap plastic plate. I brought the fork to my nose and smelled it. There was a plastic scent, as well as a hint of old salsa. I looked closely at the tomato chunk sliding down the side of the meat slice. It immediately made my stomach queasy, and I ran to the bathroom.

Nothing came up. I just stared at the empty toilet, the water sitting inside like a stagnant pond, a brownish ring smeared on the porcelain around the surface. It was enough to make me gag and break up the still water with a few stringy strands of spit. I wiped my mouth with my hand and looked in the mirror at my flushed face. There were a handful of small fresh pimples rising out from my cheeks and a large boil swelling beneath the skin of my chin.

Could it be? I wondered aloud as I undressed, needing to rinse off the nausea of the chicken bite and the memory of the dirty toilet into the shower. I noticed a small vein on the side of my left breast in the mirror as I opened the cabinet for a new bar of soap. I didn't remember the vein being there before. I was sure that it was new, another sign that I could check off on my list of possible pregnancy symptoms.

"One more day," I reminded myself, as I adjusted the water temperature to lukewarm. The next day would officially be 29 days since my last period. I added *Stop by Rite-Aid after work tomorrow for a pregnancy test* to my mental to-do list. In my mind, I was already going through the alphabetical email listings of my friends, trying to decide how I would word my exciting announcement.

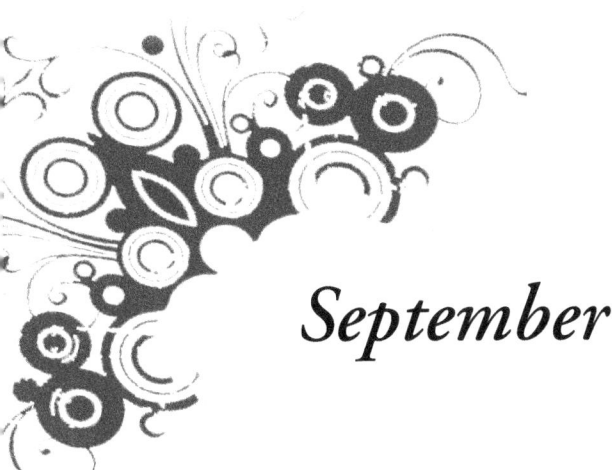

September

No. I looked down in disbelief at my underwear. NO. It couldn't be. I stared at the blood for over a minute, hoping it would go into rewind mode and climb back into my body. There had to be some other explanation. I did everything by the book. I was exhibiting all the tell tale signs.

I called my husband at the auto body shop to tell him. He responded with a quick, "Sorry, sweetie, we'll try again." That was it. No band-aids or hugs through the phone, just the sound of the sander in the background.

It wasn't enough. I didn't want *again*. I wanted *now*, with its certainty of nine more months and a list of appointments to make in my Franklin planner. I wanted him to say he would fix it, no matter how late he had to stay up on the internet to research it. I wanted him to tell me that I just forgot to flick the right switch and if I did it right then, everything would return to how it was five minutes ago.

"It's okay," he added.

"That's it?" I snapped. "That's all you have to say?"

"What do you want me to say?" he asked, his voice becoming slightly defensive.

"Nothing. You don't have to say anything," I muttered and slammed the phone back into the cradle. I was so mad at him that I could barely breathe. He had no idea what I was feeling. He was not even trying to understand that I was already walking on the slippery edge of infertility. He did not know what it felt like to be living in my body. He couldn't see my uterus, lined with crumbling gray rocks, or my ovaries, pinched closed at the sides of their thin, fragile seams.

~

"I was just so surprised that it happened the first month that we tried," one of the pregnant women in my office confessed in the hallway outside of my cubicle.

"Me, too," the voice of the other pregnant woman replied. "Are you glowing? My husband says I'm glowing." I could hear her pause as she waited for a compliment to return her way.

I didn't have to see the women to visualize their designer maternity outfits, their hands poised at their waists like there were golden Oscar awards growing inside their bellies. I wanted to go to the bathroom to throw up, and it wasn't because I was pregnant.

I wondered how I had ended up at this point, eavesdropping on two women who felt they were as entitled to their easy and comfortable pregnancies as they were to their Nordstrom credit cards. I wondered how I was still working at this school fundraising job as well. The past year had been a blur: buying an old fixer-upper in the country, getting married, quitting my teaching job, temping for the summer, and weeks of counting fliers and licking envelopes for the fundraising company.

It was not what I had pictured I would be doing when I tried to start a family. I had imagined myself lounging on a woven wood chair in a serene pasture in the English countryside, my hand wrapped around a quill pen as I finished the notes for my third best seller, a swarm of butterflies hovering in the distance, and a collie curled up at my side. My husband would be working in our moss-covered cottage, a gingery roast cooking in the hot oven, waiting with open arms for my return as he was barely able to contain his excitement over the inspirational verse dripping from my recent pages.

Instead, I looked down at the pile of school phone numbers that I still had left to call, the names of fundraising chair people listed like a generic class roster. Our receptionist called back to let me know that my husband had left a message that he would not be home until late, due to a pension meeting after work, and he needed me to pick up some Tums for him on the way home.

Line two rang and one of my top chair people, an athletic director, started a windy tirade on the other end, but I missed most of what he was saying because I was listening to one of the pregnant women confessing, "And wouldn't you know it, I haven't had a second of morning sickness. In fact, I have more energy than I have ever had in my life. I love being pregnant!"

~

The commercial said that they had helped thousands of couples conceive, so I found myself smack dab in the middle of *that section* at the local Rite Aid. *That section* was the aisle labeled *Feminine care*, and all of the items in this aisle were either blue or pink, as if those colors could disguise the odors and discharges that the products were intended to hide.

I tiptoed through the aisle, remembering when I looked out for past high school classmates or my former piano teacher, anyone who might see me choosing the Super Size tampons, or worse yet, a neighbor who might catch me buying a box of condoms and tell my mother. The ovulation kits were shelved between feminine anti-itch creams and the douches. There were four brands that were all around the same price. Two of the brands came in light blue boxes, with soft airy circles swirling behind the lettering. The other two brands had pink boxes with white lines striping the background in candy cane patterns.

I needed to choose, either blue or pink. That was when I realized I would have to expose my preference for either a boy or a girl, though no one would know except for the check out clerk and her scanner as she zapped the bar code and sent the information straight to the Pregnancy Intelligence Center housed in some remote location of the United States. I had the choice: Should I pick *blue*, with its allure of denim overalls and tree forts, or should I choose *pink*, with its closet full of dresses, hair bows, and patent leather shoes? I closed my eyes and let my fingers venture forward, my hands moving apart like opposing magnets.

~

Once I got the ovulation kit home, it took me over an hour to understand the directions. The flow charts and graphs reminded me too much of geometry class, and I was left with the same blank expression on my face, realizing that my fertile time was as hard to predict as a twelve step proof.

I translated enough of the small print to know that I needed to pee on the indicator stick included in the kit, and that a dark blue line would appear on the stick when I was in my *fertile time*. There was an asterisk and a warning at the end of the pamphlet. The small print stated that a *light* blue line could mean that fertility was *hours* or *days* away.

My stick came up a murky blue, neither light nor dark blue. I had no idea what that meant or what I should do. The directions didn't mention anything about a medium blue line. It didn't take me long to realize that I had just spent thirty bucks on a bottle of snake oil. There was no guarantee for a bouncing bundle of joy in this box, no foolproof formula or definite equation. There was only a white stick and a blue line that was the color of a hazy sky, and the set of directions that I had already torn up into little pieces and stuffed into the wastebasket. I was in between the answers, a *greater than* sign paused on my right side, a *less than* sign lurking to my left.

~

I had heard that your breasts get sore when you are pregnant, so I pressed mine until they hurt, noting every nodule and groove beneath the skin. Luckily, I was pretty flat to begin with, so it was easy to feel my ribs hidden underneath, the bones I hadn't traced with such precision since puberty.

And suddenly I was a high school girl again in my upstairs bedroom, exploring a body that took its cues from some source outside of me, pressing my breasts together so that they would create forced cleavage down the center of my chest, a sight so completely sexy that I knew it would always be out of my reach.

Then it hit me that I should lay off the pressure because somewhere under there were milk ducts, or at least that is what I had heard, though nothing I was touching felt anything like a food source.

The boys laughed two rows behind me as the science teacher circled the breasts with his purple marker on the overhead projector.

"The breasts contain milk ducts," the teacher explained, "for feeding," and I drew bulbous roots growing all over the chest of my sketched female torso, wild shrubbery that climbed over her entire upper body.

"I'd sure like to drink them!" one boy shouted from behind me.

"Do they come with chocolate syrup?" another one chimed in.

The boys' jokes were loud enough for the whole class to hear. I can assume now that the teacher did hear them, though he chose to pretend he did not due to the weight of another long day of no air conditioning and an itchy tie against his throat. The rest of the class and I stayed busy copying the correct spelling of ducts and mammary glands onto our papers. I suddenly felt very self conscious and hunched my shoulders together to hide my own breasts through the rest of that seventh period, though they were already strapped down tight in a Double A sized bra.

~

I was pregnant with my mother in the dream, only she was not a fetus, but a miniature copy of herself—like one of the people in The Borrowers books that I always picked to read for my extra credit reports.

She was pointing the right direction for me to walk, and I could see the imprint of her long index finger moving back and forth inside my stomach. I followed her guide, turning left around a prickly holly tree, and then jumping over a loose telephone cable when her finger quickly jutted up into my ribs. She knew the way better than I did, even though I was the one who could see and move my feet.

"Slow down," her voice muffled through the tiny fold in the middle of my belly button.

"Okay," I said, realizing I had been going too fast. She could not keep her glasses from falling off of her face. There was not enough elbow room in my stomach for her to keep pushing them back up onto the bridge of her nose.

"I'll try to slow down," I told her, but she didn't reply to my remark.

"Mom?" I said, hoping I would feel a finger or toe poking in response. My belly remained motionless. I couldn't tell if she was still inside me.

"Mom!" I screamed, but there was nothing, and I suddenly felt more alone than I had ever felt by myself.

~

"They blessed four babies at church today," my mother announced during one of our weekly Sunday evening dinners at my parents' house. My mother was the only one who still attended church in the family. My father had never become a member of any church, though his beliefs tended to lean towards his Primitive Baptist roots. My mother had converted to Mormonism about the time that she and my father had married, leading to a life of religious differences and arguments.

"Wow. Four," I said, pretending to be excited.

"I think you went to Sunday school with two of the mothers," she said, turning towards me as she passed her broccoli and chicken casserole.

I faintly remembered the women she named. They were girls the last time I saw them, seventh graders with retainers and jelly bracelets. I was twelve when I finally refused to put on a skirt and dress shoes and accompany my mother and my sister to the Mormon Church in Towson. Instead, I stayed home with my father, watching Laurel and Hardy movies and eating dry Lucky Charms cereal. My sister was still young enough for bribery, my mother never mentioning the Roy Rogers bags carefully stuffed under the seats of the car after they came home.

I knew I should have been happy for the other pregnant women. I didn't want to be jealous, but I couldn't help feeling angry at their precious rewards for staying at church, for waiting to have sex until they were married and keeping cigarettes and alcohol at arm's length. These girls had stayed on the good list, and were handed healthy children like deserved presents, while I, on the other hand, was doomed to stay on the bad list, a mile long tainted scroll of poor choices highlighted in yellow marker. I was surely going to receive at least a week of infertility for each beer that I had sucked down and a day of struggle for every curse word that had passed through my lips.

"They don't seem old enough to have kids," I remarked, picturing the girls' fluorescent pink over the shoulder sweatshirts and matching hair bows at the last mixer I remembered attending, Madonna and Michael Jackson specifically barred from the DJ's play list.

"But they are the same age as you are," my mother pointed out, passing the casserole across the table to my pale sister.

~

The pastel drawings in the Mormon storybook had sketches romantic enough to mesmerize the attention of any child, especially one who often found herself staring at the dusty ridge between the orange industrial carpet and the portable wall of her Sunday school classroom.

One of the pictures showed a huge line of children waiting in heaven for their parental assignments. God stood like the supreme teacher at the entry gates, looking over each child before searching his list for the appropriate choice. The children looked like they were getting ready to burst through the gates of a carnival: their hands reaching up in excitement, their bodies pushing forward, just waiting for the ticket booth to open. All of the children wore airy white garments that puffed out above their bare feet like clouds and made them look like little angels. They were all waiting for their turn, for God to give them the signal to start their journeys down into their earth parents' arms.

Our Sunday school teacher held the book on her knees and we took turns approaching her, looking at each individual child until we found one that we resembled. It took me awhile, but I finally found myself 64th in the line. I was the blond girl with two ponytails almost hidden behind a chubby boy with a cowlick in the front of his hair. I was glad that I was in the middle of the line, so I could watch the other children go before me and know the best way to spread my arms.

Our teacher told us we had each personally selected our parents, and that we had chosen them for very special reasons. I tried to imagine what my parents were doing when I first saw them from heaven. I pictured the yellowing print from their pre-children photo album: my parents in the living room of what would become my childhood home, scratching the stomach of their new beagle puppy, my father winking to the forgotten photographer lining up the shot from the hallway. It felt reassuring to know that I had picked them to be my parents, and that my arrival at their house was not an accident. I took pride in the fact that I had carefully plotted my course from heaven to Dance Mill Road.

Could there actually be a child up there waiting for me? I couldn't imagine what child would want to choose me after seeing the way I cried in the shower and ignored the dead mice that the cat left on the front porch. What child would find comfort in a house full of dust balls and burnt toast?

It was much more frightening to be on this other side of the journey. I had to be the strong one this time. No one would be there to catch me. I had to be ready if a child fell, like an unexpected rain, from the sky.

~

It was time. I was ready. I took a big breath.

I started slowly, unscrewing the gold ball from the top and pulling the silver hook through the bottom hole. I could feel the metal resisting, caught on the last inch of my skin. After one last tug, the ring was out, leaving the skin around my belly button puckered and red. The holes looked awkward and lacking, like my stomach was missing its glasses or its familiar set of bushy eyebrows. From far away, the holes could have been two bite marks, two sores left from the fleeting beast called *my twenties*.

I screwed the gold ball back onto the hook and placed the ring in the soap dish in the bathroom. The specimen was now removed, and with it, the last physical proof of any fading rebellion.

I moved my hand over my belly, wiping the scars with orange antibacterial soap, and closed my eyes to see if I could feel any trace of the holes. There was hardly any difference; my fingertips slid over my belly button in one smooth stroke. My stomach was an empty plane now, a blank piece of paper.

"Okay," I told myself, "There is room now."

I took the belly ring and dried it on a clean towel. The gold shined, and for a second I didn't want to lock it away in the bottom drawer of my jewelry box, next to my first lost tooth and a love letter from my ninth grade boyfriend.

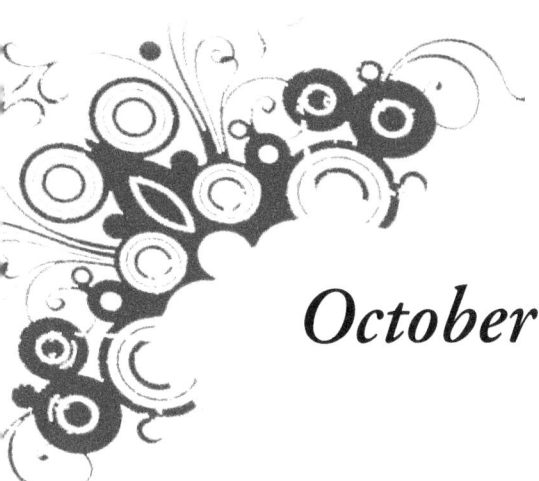

October

"Which way do I turn it?" I asked my husband before attempting to find the SET button on the clock.

"Spring forward, Fall back," he mumbled, already slipping into the hard sleep I have only dreamed about in my insomnia filled life.

"Fall back," I whispered and continued to hold the hour button down until it made its way back around to the p.m. numbers.

My husband had been reluctant to keep up the sex marathon, so it had been another uneventful night in the bedroom. I was happy to stay in my flannel pajamas with the cold starting to creep in through the window cracks. I tightened the drawstring around the waist of my pajama bottoms, knowing they would stay that way until the sun broke through the dusty shades the next morning.

My plans of pregnancy seemed completely absurd at that moment. I didn't know who I was fooling, actually thinking that conception would just happen at the drop of a dime. I patted the bed and the dogs came running in. I moved over enough so that they could jump up and squeeze in between my husband and me. Within five minutes, both dogs and my husband were snoring, and I was still wide-awake.

"Fall back," I told myself, as I re-adjusted my body into a side curl. I wanted to cry, but I couldn't. There wasn't room with everyone sleeping next to me and the house continuing with its usual creaking. I wanted to sleep, to forget about my longing, but I kept looking at the clock and trying to figure out what time it actually was, and what time it would actually be the next day, and the next week, and the next month when my ovulation cycle would start all over again.

~

I was two hours late. It had been exactly twenty-eight days and two hours since my last period, and I was already in Rite Aid, debating over which pregnancy test to buy. I decided to opt for the one that was on sale, the generic brand with the words *Two Tests Included* written in big purple letters on its box. I casually placed my purchase on the register counter, paid with my credit card, and made a mad dash back to my car.

The cold air of the parking lot seemed to be drawing attention to my secret as a light breeze crinkled the bag, and I felt like I was about to be caught at any moment. With the pregnancy test jostling inside the plastic bag, I was no longer undercover and inconspicuous. It was too obvious that I was on my way to an arranged date, an upcoming threesome: the car, the pregnancy test, and me.

Back in the safety of the car, I peeled the tight plastic wrap from around the box and took the test out. I was careful not to raise it above window level, just in case there was video surveillance from the strip mall. I immediately stuffed the test into my purse and checked twice in the rearview mirror to make sure no one had spotted me. The only movement that I could see was an old Baltimore *City Paper* blowing across the parking spot behind me.

As I pulled out of the parking lot, the reality of my infidelity hit me. I couldn't go home, not where the dogs, the stained carpet, and the ringing phone would all know what I was doing. It needed to be a secret rendezvous. I needed to find another place to take the test.

Taco Bell was the first place that I sighted with a public restroom. The restroom door was locked, so I had to wait in the dingy front hallway while I heard the toilet flush, followed by the sink running for over ten minutes. I shifted my weight back and forth from each foot, pretending to look like I had to use the bathroom. I reached into my purse and touched the test to make sure that it was still there. The water finally stopped running, and then the automatic hand dryer came on.

I couldn't wait much longer. My nerves were already pulsing on their ends. The glass entry door kept opening and closing and opening and the customers continued to dribble in, giving me suspicious glances before lining up before the registers. The hallway lights flickered and I looked up to notice a pile of dead bugs caught inside one of the plastic covers. The hand dryer cut off, and I breathed a sigh of relief before it started right back up again.

Finally, after what seemed like hours, the lock released and the door swung open. An older woman shuffled out with light blue tinted hair and love handles the size of small countries. She squeezed by me, and I rushed into the restroom, overwhelmed by the scent of Aqua Net Hairspray and Lysol.

~

The pink line was so faint that I had to tilt the stick to the left in the sick green light of the restroom to see it. I yanked the instructions out of the box and skimmed through them until I found a section that confirmed a faint line represented a very early pregnancy.

I couldn't help but wonder if I had accidentally picked up someone else's pregnancy test. Did it really show a pink line? Perhaps the test belonged to another woman, a tired woman already gray with worry and age. I could hear her exhausted voice as she threatened her three children to stay in the backseat of their minivan with the doors locked while she ran inside the fast food restroom. Or, maybe a frightened fourteen year old left it, after her best friend urged her to abandon the evidence before her mother found it. Either way, I could see the woman and the girl, their anxious faces, the curves of their wrists as they flushed the toilet and slowly walked out of the stall and into their new lives. However, I couldn't see myself, looking down at this thin white stick, trying to find the right angle of light to be sure that my eyes weren't fooling me.

At any moment I knew the door would fly open, and a Taco Bell employee would come marching in, a piece of cheese dangling from her lips. She would grab the test from my hands as if I had stolen her purse and then push me down onto the dirty tile. I would be too caught off guard to react, her stinging words leaving me shivering on the bathroom floor: *That was mine. Who do you think you are? Quit taking what isn't yours!*

~

I congratulated myself for coming up with the adorable idea of wrapping up the pregnancy stick as my husband's early birthday present. My hands shook as I rummaged through the wrapping paper box until I found a silver gift bag that wasn't too beaten up. I pulled off the attached tag which read, *Happy Birthday, Love Mom and Dad*, and tried to straighten out a couple of the wrinkles. We were out of tissue paper, so I lined the top of the bag with twenty staples in aesthetic exchange. I pictured the pregnancy stick, all by itself in the white interior of the bag, with only the two pink lines to provide any color or comfort against the cold blankness. Would it will be able to breathe with all of the air stapled out? I didn't want the test to suffocate and lose its light pink line from a lack of oxygen.

I paced the floor until my husband called. He said that he would be home as soon as he finished a serpentine belt replacement. I hung up the phone and turned on *Inside Edition* to try to distract myself. The longer I sat the more I felt like I held the pass code to a nuclear reactor. Someone else had to know. What if something happened to me before my husband came home? What if my house exploded, or I suddenly died of a brain aneurysm? No one would ever have known that I was pregnant. I bit my thumbnail down until the skin started to bleed. I debated about writing the words, *I am pregnant*, with the date, on a piece of paper as a precaution while the sun faded behind the beige curtains. The traffic began to break down from a constant hum to individual motors coming and going.

My husband walked in a little after seven, yelled at the dogs for barking too loud, and dropped his wallet, four receipts, and a pile of change onto the coffee table.

"Hey," I said, knowing he had to notice the fluctuation in my voice, the way my pupils were dilated to the size of quarters.

"I was stuck doing oil changes all morning," he complained.

"And to top it off," he continued, "a crazy lady came in after lunch and accused us of stealing a bottle of Windex from her glove compartment."

I sat and listened to the rest of his day's disappointments, picturing one of the lot boys smuggling the sky blue bottle into the pocket of his baggy jeans before hiding it in his trunk, on top of a pile of old CDs and beer cans.

"Did anyone take it?" I asked.

"What?" he asked.

"The Windex?"

"No," my husband snapped, "We found it in her center console."

As his tirade ended, he walked out of the living room and started to head to his basement get-away, otherwise known as the man pit.

Okay. Do it now, I tried to convince myself.

Do it before it gets too dark, before the daylight is gone. I was suddenly completely aware that the light would make it easier for me to open my mouth. I would be able to look out the window as I talked, to latch my gaze onto the rooster weathervane above our shed. My words would not know where to go in the dark. They would be scattered like lost children in the air.

"Wait, um, first I want to give you your birthday present," I blurted out in one quick breath.

"But my birthday isn't until next week," he said, turning around from the top of the basement steps.

Without responding, I ran into the bedroom to get the gift bag before I changed my mind about telling him.

When I returned to the living room, he was sitting on the couch, his bare feet propped up on the coffee table. I handed him the bag without a word. He popped the staples apart in one quick rip and reached in. He pulled out the stick, looked at it for a second, and then squinted his eyes at me.

"Does this mean?" he asked.

"Yep." I said, rolling my bottom lip into my mouth and sinking my upper teeth down into it until it stung.

I forced myself to look into his face, to see if his response would make it feel more real, but I couldn't read his expression. His eyes were blank.

Then a raw smile started to spread across his face, the kind I hadn't seen in years, not since 1980, when my little sister ran into the living room on Christmas morning to find a new pink bike leaning against the prickly needles of the tree, its silver streamers cascading from the handle bars like artificial water fountains.

"Let's wait until I go to the doctor to let people know," I said.

Fifteen minutes later my parents, my sister, and the six friends of ours who were home knew the news. I smothered them with questions:

Do you think it will be a girl or a boy?

Do you think it will have my slanted eyes, my double jointed elbows, or my husband's flat feet?

Do you think it will like to write poetry or to work on carburetors?

Their answers blurred together. I wasn't listening anyway. I was just talking. My mouth was going a mile a minute, and it wouldn't stop.

"Do you think we should do the nursery in yellow?" I asked my mother.

"Um. If you want to," she said, and then asked me when I was going to the doctor.

"Oh, I haven't scheduled it yet."

"Wow. Things sure have changed," she replied.

Her voice sounded distant, hesitant, and a little reluctant.

"Aren't you thrilled to become a grandparent?" I asked, waiting for the exuberant response I knew just had to be coming.

"Sure," she said, somewhat less dramatically than I had expected, as if I had just asked her if she liked canned pears or cottage cheese. "It will be great."

"It will be great!" my little sister mimicked sarcastically in the background before slamming her bedroom door and turning up Marilyn Manson so loud I could barely make out my mother's "Gotta go" and "Goodbye."

By the end of the night, it felt like I had known about the pregnancy for six weeks instead of six hours. I stayed up late, just in case one of the friends who wasn't home wanted to return my subtle message, "Call me back for some really big news!"

However, the phone and the computer stayed silent and the usual Thursday night television shows were all repeats, so I was left looking up at the ceiling above my bed and petting the dogs. They whimpered and scratched themselves and didn't seem to notice that anything had changed.

~

Even from my pillow, I could see it stuffed into my bookshelf; the thick spine caught between *Latin: Lessons for the Beginner* and *The New Our Bodies, Ourselves*. I hadn't touched *Moby Dick* since I had purchased it for an American Literature course in college and then dropped the class after the schedule interfered with my bookstore job at Hunt Valley Mall. I could see the middle of the whale on the spine, a gray mass cutting through the green sky of the dense paperback. A harpooner was paused in mid-throw, his spear sharp enough to burrow into the whale's dark rubbery skin.

The book always looked so ominous to me, so unbreakable, though I never admitted it to my fellow English majors. Of course, I pieced together enough information through class discussions to learn the themes of struggle and obsession, the captain's need to hunt for finality beyond his actual duty. I even remembered enough of my teacher's references to answer the GRE analogy correctly: "Captain Ahab is to _____ as addict is to drug. However, I always knew that I was a fake English major, pretending to have a vast library inside my head when all I had was a shelf full of Stephen King and Dean Koontz books.

Read me, the book called from the warped shelf, and suddenly it made sense to start two journeys, a physical one and a literary one. I pulled the book out and straightened the bent corner of its cover. The rowers were keeping their small boat steady among the spray and curling waves, while the sea gulls circled the volcanic jet of the whale's spout. The whaling ship waited in the background, just watching as coal smoked from its thick belly and rose up into the sky.

I opened the first page.

"Call me Ishmael," it began, just as I expected it to begin.

"Are you going to read for awhile?" my husband came into the bedroom and asked, just as I expected him to.

"No, just this chapter," I said, and return to "Loomings," and Ishmael's first steps towards his new life at sea.

~

I felt like I was impersonating someone when the words came out: "I'm pregnant, and I need to schedule an appointment." I was in my car, calling my gynecologist's office from my cell phone outside my office building. I had decided not to tell my boss until I went to the doctor. It was five minutes before I was supposed to be at my desk, getting ready to organize the next set of high school fundraising kick-offs.

The nurse had to be on to me. She had to know that this was a prank call, and I was getting ready to laugh and hang up the phone. I was actually surprised when I heard the sound of her turning the pages of an appointment book.

"How about next Friday," she said, tapping her pen in the column for next Friday.

"Sure," I coughed. "Next Friday's fine."

"How about 9:30?"

"That's fine," I managed, and then stuttered out my name and phone number.

"Okay. We'll see you then," she said.

I mustered up a "thanks" and pressed the END key to finish the call.

"Next Friday. 9:30," I whispered aloud, and then realized I had already scheduled a kick-off for the next Friday at 10:00. I looked at the one story industrial building in front of me and knew there was nothing else left for me to do but to lie.

"Hi," I tentatively said, as I hobbled into my boss's office and sat down in one of the stiff orange chairs in front of his desk.

"I really hurt my back this weekend. I called my doctor, and he wants me to take it easy. He wants me to come in to see him next Friday at 9:30, that's the only open slot, but I have a kick off scheduled for that day. Could you do it for me?" My boss flinched and started to squirm in his seat. He hated speaking in public, especially in front of large groups of high school kids.

"Don't worry. The kids won't throw anything at you," I laughed, picturing my nervous and bald forty-year-old boss up on the school auditorium stage, trying to explain the fundraiser to an auditorium full of smelly and pimply freshmen.

"Ah," my boss hesitated, "Sure. Just let me know if you need help with any of your deliveries." He had bought it.

"Boy, my back used to go out all the time when I worked at Caldor," he reminisced, and started into a saga about his health problems while working at Caldor, the discount department store near Belvedere that had closed over a decade ago. I pretended to grimace in pain and adjusted my seating position as he recounted five years of early morning loading dock nightmares.

"Here, let me help you up," he said after snapping back into the present.

"Thanks," I smiled; after all, I had killed two birds with one stone.

~

The pregnancy stick was buried deep within the zippered part of my purse, the same place where I used to hide my birth control pills when I lived at home. I had already snuck forty-seven peeks to confirm that the two lines were visible, and that was still not enough for me to believe that the two lines were permanent, that one of them had not faded away into the darkness of my purse.

I drew two lines throughout the day to remind myself that it was real. I made two thin lines with a blue marker on the left hand side of my shipping invoices. I consciously dipped my finger into the leftover spaghetti sauce from lunch and drew two red lines down the center of my napkin. All of the payment-return envelopes that I mailed out had two black ink lines, purposeful smudges I had produced by pushing them too far into the postage machine. It was my secret code; my binary language that would go unnoticed under all passing eyes.

The lines were two lives, the two people it took to make this pregnancy, the two people who were now taking up my one body. I made the lines parallel, one for each of my hands, two short sticks that had been sanded down into two smooth handles. They were my two grips, the only holds that I could grasp for safety. I clung onto them with desperation, without a trainer, or even a spotter for that matter.

~

There was barely room for me to squeeze onto my mother's lap as she took the Fisher Price stethoscope out of the plastic doctor's box and carefully placed the ear tips into my ears.

"Let's try here," she said, holding the plastic chest piece to her hard belly. I tried to listen, to hear something that sounded like the baby she had told me was growing inside, a little baby sister who would need me to show her how to tie her shoes and put the knife next to the fork at the kitchen table.

"Do you hear anything?" my mother's voice echoed through the ear tips, and I jumped, taken off guard by the deep beat of her voice. She sounded like she was inside my head, tunneling down into the hidden canals of my ears.

"It's just amplifying the sound," she explained, stroking my long braid with her hand. "See?" She held the chest piece up for me to examine.

I tapped the pink spongy bottom of the chest piece with my finger. Crackly thumps filled my ears.

"The sound goes through there and becomes louder when it hits your ears. It's just like the one Mommy's doctor uses, only it isn't quite as strong," she said.

"Let's try it again. Okay?" I nodded, and she held my hand to her stomach, the chest piece filling my entire palm. We sat in silence for a few seconds, and then I grew impatient.

"Does she know we are listening for her?" I asked.

"I'm not sure," my mother replied. "She might be able to feel the heat from

your hand."

"*I think she knows,*" I smiled. "She knows I'm her sister. She can just tell. You know, the way I've always known that you are my mother."

~

I kept waiting for the curtain to close, for the time to run out before anyone had guessed my word. I was making the mental image: holding my hands out in a wide loop around my belly, walking back and forth like a bow-legged horse rider. Still, no one could guess the word, an eight-letter word written on a white strip of paper that I had pulled out of a hat over a week ago. They could only see my flat stomach, the clothes that fit the same as they did before. There was no way to act out the uneasiness living inside my body. I opened my eyes as wide as I could and pointed down at my belly with my chin, attempting to project the word telepathically. I could feel the word trying to escape from the cage of my teeth.

"A bloated lady," someone yelled from the front row.

"A sick person," another voice hollered from the orchestra pit.

"The Emperor in his new clothes," a third guess bellowed from the balcony.

My turn was almost up; my hourglass was almost out of sand. I could see the next player watching me from the side of the stage, a shorter strip of white paper curled inside her hand. I only had a few seconds left.

Pregnant! Pregnant! I wanted to scream, but my mouth had to stay shut, since that is how the game is played.

~

"Everything looks fine," my doctor said when we were back in his office. "We'll schedule you for your first set of blood work when you leave." He pulled a small paper wheel out of his desk that looked like a tip percentage chart.

"Let's see. When was your last period?" he asked.

I told him, and he turned the top layer of the paper wheel around the lower wheel until the date lined up in the cut out window.

"June 25th," he concluded, and looked back up at me. "Congratulations."

"Thanks," I responded, caught off guard with this simple method for determining such a momentous date.

"Did you have any questions?" he asked.

I pulled the list out of my pocket and began taking notes.

"Are there any dietary restrictions?" I started off, holding my pen like an eager reporter.

"Just be sensible," he chuckled, "No alcohol, of course, and limit your caffeine intake."

I scribbled, "Be sensible," next to my first question and proceeded to the next one.

"What about sex? Is it safe?"

"Yes," he smiled, "it's safe, as long as you're not having any bleeding or cramping."

"No-- bleeding, cramping," I quickly jotted down.

"When do I get the first ultrasound?" I asked, already anxious to picture the baby on the ultrasound screen, mouthing "Hi, Mommy" back to me with its tiny lips.

There was a knock on the door. The nurse popped her head in.

"Sorry to bother you, Doctor, but there's a patient who really needs to speak to you on the phone."

"Excuse me," my doctor said and picked up the phone that was attached to the wall. I could hear a woman's voice, high-pitched and erratic, coming through the receiver.

I looked down at my list and the answers that I had scribbled. My notes were so messy that I knew I would have to recopy them when I got home. I retraced my answers with my pen while the phone call continued.

"It sounds like it might be," he calmly stated into the phone. The woman's voice became louder. I could hear uncontrolled sobbing on the other end.

"It happens," he finally interrupted the caller. "Why don't you come in as soon as you can?" I heard a slight whimper come through the receiver, and then there was dead silence. He put the phone down and smiled. "Sorry about that. What was your last question?"

~

It was a long time away, a due date that hung at the end of the school year, a day for which all of our neighborhood kids would be holding their breath. I looked at the free calendar from the local hardware store hanging on my kitchen wall and the current month of *October* with its picture of the four-foot tall pumpkin from Valley View Farms. I flipped past *November* and its recipe for Aunt Cookie's oyster stuffing, and lingered on *December*, with the Long Green Volunteer Fire Company Santa Claus smiling from the side window of a green fire truck. I couldn't imagine what I might look like at that point. Would I have a pudgy stomach? Would I be past this stage of fear and uncertainty, my pregnancy finally visible in a secure warm ball?

I licked my thumb and breezed past *January*, with its diagram of the different retail cuts of beef, a cartoon cow sliced and labeled into preferential portions. Would *February's* recommended storage periods for cornstarch, dry yeast, and vinegar find me in the midst of my second trimester? Would I be able to feel the baby kicking by the time I reached *March's* photo of the hardware store owner's six month old grandson propped up on the seat of an old John Deere? Would we be setting up the nursery during *April's* Helpful Household Hints by Pastor Evans?

I ran my finger along the Equivalent Measurements Guide for the month of *May*, the month when I would probably feel like I was about to burst. Then I was finally at *June*, my due date month, and I placed my finger on June 25. The block was blank, nestled in mid-way through the fourth week. That couldn't be right. There was nothing special about this square. I knew that if I had closed my eyes and thrown a dart, it never would have ended up here, on this random space printed below a picture of the Glen Arm Lion's Club, the aging men's arms raised in yet another outdated toast.

~

I repeated the pregnancy rules in my head. They were my new guidelines, my *Ten Commandments* that I had found in one of my pregnancy books:

1. *No smoking*
2. *No drinking*
3. *No drugs*
4. *No x-rays*
5. *No unpasteurized cheese*
6. *No whirlpools or saunas*
7. *No changing cat liter boxes*
8. *No raw meat or raw fish*
9. *No exposure to paint fumes*
10. *No heavy lifting*

I thought it would feel natural to follow the pregnancy rules. I thought my body would automatically be disgusted by the thought of a beer or a big glass of Sangria. Instead, I found myself overly interested in the forbidden. My office mate's extra large cups of Dunkin' Donuts coffee smiled at me with their morning wake up calls. I found myself envying my next door neighbor out in the whirlpool on his deck, his coarse chest hair hovering above the frothy bubbles. Even the sauna at the gym lured my feet extra close to its wooden door, the heat climbing over my toes, pulling at my ankles with its alluring warmth. I thought there would be some internal stop sign, some way to keep myself from going astray, from endangering the baby that I was carrying. But there wasn't a thing, just my own responsibility to say *no*. There was no physical line of danger, and I needed an actual line, like the one my mother would draw down the middle of the backseat of our station wagon. I needed the reassurance of my familiar threat to my sister: *If you cross this line you will die!*

~

The planets are not lined up, at least that is what my mother said when I told her that it felt like the world was out of focus and all of the floors were tilted.

"It always feels strange at the beginning," she explained, "especially when it's your first one."

I had nothing to compare to, so I tried to convince myself that it was normal to want to cry every other minute. I told myself that all pregnant women were overwhelmed and exhausted and at least half of them felt like they couldn't manage another early morning of shampoo and conditioner.

My planets had to be completely out of order because I couldn't even focus enough to remember to put deodorant under both arms. The car, too, seemed out of my reach of control, almost drifting into the garage after I fumbled for the brake when I forgot to shift the gear back into park.

My planets had also caused me to knock one of my boss's inspirational plaques off his desk when he was in the lunchroom. The glass cracked across the exclamation at the top, *You are the only one who makes life happen!* and I re-positioned it behind another plaque with the quote, *Strive for Excellence,* hoping that he wouldn't notice. It only took about five minutes after he returned from lunch before I heard his condemning voice traveling down the hall: "Who broke my plaque?" I pretended to be counting book returns, moving my finger down and across each stack of books like a serious inventory taker.

My planets had to be spinning too fast. Maybe their rings were starting to disintegrate. Maybe there was a meteor headed straight for their course, ready to knock them all down like bowling pins. Whatever the scientific explanation, it definitely felt like something was wrong. It felt like something bad was about to go down.

~

It was just the bathroom, the bloody toilet tissue, and me. I could hear the Halloween party continuing on the other side of the door, as if nothing had changed, as if I had not stepped into the bathroom with the orange and black candles and the framed playbill of *Rent* positioned perfectly straight above the towel ring. The voices sounded a hundred miles away. I couldn't separate the different pitches or the tones. I couldn't tell which laughter belonged to the hostess, dressed as a Geisha, and which one was coming from the naughty nurse I had just been talking to before I suddenly felt wet and excused myself to the bathroom. All of the sounds blurred into one block of noise, which hung like a thick fog on the other side of the door.

The wooden door separated me from the party and the woman I was before I entered into the bathroom. The door might as well have been made of steel, as the weight of going back into the party felt just as impassable. I didn't know if I had the ability to persuade my body into cooperating, and I didn't know if I could muster up enough strength to keep from falling apart in front of everyone.

With my pantyhose still down around my ankles and my long black skirt sitting in a puddle on the floor, I procrastinated the inevitable by examining my Olive Oil wig in the mirror and tried to smooth down my own frizzy hairs, which were creeping out from the front of the wig.

I reluctantly stuffed a ball of toilet paper into my underwear and pulled my pantyhose up over my hips. After my skirt was on, I flushed the red water down the toilet and slowly pushed the door open into the rec room full of drunken revelers.

I was suddenly the new student at school, trying to find a spot at one of the crowded cafeteria tables. The partygoers didn't miss a beat in their current conversations. They didn't even know that I had just slipped out to use the bathroom, or that I had found bad news waiting for me on the top of the toilet tissue like a foreshadowing black spot.

I hated all of them at that moment. Their costumes were ridiculous and petty, their voices loud and irritating. I saw a cowgirl point to a small scab on her shoulder. The cowgirl's boyfriend, in matching cowboy attire, hit the bull's eye of the dartboard and congratulated himself because no one else was watching. Two KISS members practiced air guitar in the corner. They didn't recognize the freedom in their strumming fingers or their slurred speech.

I tried to find my husband, but the house was so crammed with people that I could barely move from the doorway frame of the bathroom. I started pushing elbows out of my way, tipping over drinks, and pulling down the annoying plastic bats that were hanging from the ceiling, just low enough to brush the top of my head. I bumped past two gypsies smoking a joint and almost tripped over a Cheshire cat grinning from ear to ear in front of the sofa. Finally, I reached the kitchen and saw my husband's bare bicep, smeared with the ink from the anchor tattoo I had so carefully drawn just two hours earlier.

"We have to leave now," I yelled to him over the music that someone had just cranked up to window breaking capacity. He opened up the refrigerator and scanned the two bottom shelves full of beer. I was sure that he was pretending not to hear me.

"What?" he replied, his hand mid-way between a Natty Bo and a Natural Light.

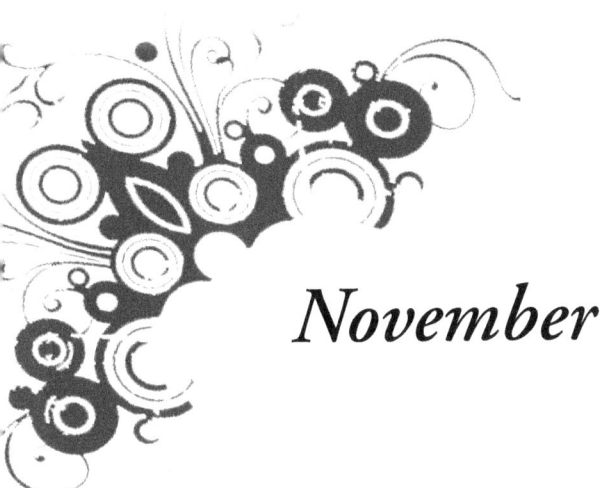

November

Spotting (Verb Transitive) 1: to stain the character or reputation of: DISGRACE 2: to mark in or with a spot: STAIN 3: to single out: IDENTIFY, esp. to note as a known criminal or a suspicious person.–Webster

"I'm bleeding," I sobbed into the phone. "I need to talk to the doctor!"

"Okay," the answering service voice responded. "I'll have the doctor call you back."

The woman's voice was steady and unemotional. She took my name and phone number, and I hung up and paced the house.

Five minutes later the phone rang. I hesitated for a moment before I picked up. My heart pounded through my chest as I brought the receiver to my ear.

"What's going on?" the doctor asked. I summarized the terrible evening and the blood that wouldn't stop.

For a moment I was worried that he was no longer on the phone, that I'd just been admitting this information to the empty air, but then I heard a light breath, and he asked me to describe the color of the blood.

"Umm," I was puzzled by his question.

"Is it brown, pink, or red?"

Suddenly I couldn't remember the exact shade. Was it bright red, the color of a new stop sign? Or was it pink, the sickening sweet hue of Barbie dolls and cotton candy? Or maybe it was brown, like the creek behind our house after a heavy rain.

I knew I was not the master of the color wheel. I knew that I could barely remember the primary colors on a good day, but I thought I could tell the difference between pink, red and brown. Whatever was happening to my hormones was also blurring my vision, and the only reasonable answer I could tell the doctor was "all of them."

I heard a slight sigh, "It might just be spotting. As long as it's brown blood, just keep an eye on it. I will schedule you for an early ultrasound, to see if the heartbeat is visible yet."

"O.K.," I said, like an obedient school girl.

"Just keep an eye on it," he repeated.

He hung up before I had enough time to tell him that I did not have enough eyes to watch out for everything — I needed at least 200 eyes to watch out for all of the things that scared me about this pregnancy.

~

This time I was back in high school in the dream, standing mid-way down the orange hallway with the rusting metal lockers. I was trying to remember the combination to my locker, to return to the clot baby I left inside, safely cushioned between my coat and my gym uniform during the long school day.

Frantically, I was trying every possible number. I turned the combination wheel to the left two times, past the number 28, and then I turned it to the right one time, past the number 16, until I reached the number 9. No luck. Next, I tried turning it to the right first, past the number 17, and then turning it to the left past the number 21. I stopped the dial on the number 12 and pulled: still nothing. The lock's shackle stayed shut tight in its warm hole. I tried birthdays, addresses, and phone numbers, any sequence that might make sense. I was panicking, my fingers sweating against the cheap silver metal of the lock.

I continued to search for the right combination while the rest of the students trickled out of the school. The lights began to dim, and the janitor started pushing his cleaning cart up the long hallway towards me. Then, all I could hear was the sound of the wet drop of his mop against the floor.

Finally, the lock gave, and I yanked the locker open to find the charred remains of a child. The clot baby was barely there; a mere flap, blackened to the color of tar. It could barely make out a breath, but there was enough of a puff for me to know that it was still alive. I held its small body in my hands.

"I will take care of you," I wanted to whisper, but I couldn't speak, I could only rock it back and forth in my cupped hands until its raw chest finally stopped rising.

~

The blond technician rolled a protective rubber sleeve over the internal ultrasound probe and slid some lubricant up and down the tip with her palm before she asked me to insert it. I took the large plastic piece and awkwardly pushed it inside of me. Once I had it in place, I nodded, and she took over the task, slightly turning the probe with her manicured hand. She was quick with her movements, twisting the probe sharply to the left, and then slowly rotating it back to the right.

I tried to keep focused on her face, which was framed like a picture between my knees. Her skin was smooth and clean, the kind of skin from an Oil of Olay commercial, without a single freckle or blemish, the kind of skin I had never had. Her hair was cut into long layers, with perfect end curls that made me want to run my fingers through them.

"Relax," I told myself, but I couldn't keep my goose-pimpled thighs from shaking. She brushed her hand against my ankle, and I looked around for the video camera that had to be filming us, for the director to crawl out from beneath the examining table, his thin mustache trimmed and freshly greased. However, the only possible hiding spot that I could see was behind the glass jar of swabs on the cabinet, and it was too transparent a choice for a real voyeur.

The technician went about her business, just another day at the office looking inside women. She didn't even flinch when I said, "It hurts," and she pulled the probe back just enough to release the pressure, like a true expert. "Right there," she purred, and I turned to look at the monitor's screen.

For all I could tell my internal ultrasound was actually displaying a gourmet appetizer of seaweed and brown sauce. There was a dark bubble running down the middle of the monitor's screen and light flecks of gray and black that kept blurring back and forth along the edges. I blinked and squinted at the screen, trying to identify any image that might resemble a pregnancy. I couldn't see a single form that looked like *life*, or a single symbol that represented *baby*.

The technician kept her right hand on the probe while she adeptly used her left hand to center the image from the keyboard under the monitor. She positioned a curser to the left of a small shadow that was nestled into the lowest point in the screen and tapped on the touch pad until a black dotted line appeared. She moved the line across the shadow and then released the curser and repeated the procedure vertically.

"I can't find a heartbeat," she said, finally breaking the long silence.

"But you are still early, and the size is within range. Some heartbeats are not visible until the end of the seventh week. We'll have to do another one then."

Before I could comprehend her sentence, she had pulled the probe out and was peeling the protective rubber sleeve off with her thumb and forefinger. The monitor stared back at me with the same sterile gray screen that I had seen when I initially walked into the examining room.

No, I wanted to tell her. *You have to go back. You have to look around just a little longer. You might have missed the heartbeat. If only you had moved the probe more to the left, we might have seen it.* Now the screen was empty, and there was not a single sign that there was ever a pregnancy, no proof that the inside of my body was once magnified into thousands of microscopic particles.

~

The doctor recommended staying off my feet and resting as much as I could. He scheduled me for another ultrasound for a week later, when the heartbeat should be visible. I took his recommendation to mean that every time I pressed the heel of my foot into the ground I was digging the baby straight into its grave. For the next week, I was aware of every step that I took, feeling the cushions of my toes trying to pry the embryo loose from my body. The pressure of the pregnancy was too much for my size 10's. They couldn't handle the constant fight against gravity, my weight automatically compressing my uterus, squeezing every tissue to the brink of rupture.

    I did what I could: I quit going to the gym, I quit lifting the laundry basket, the trashcan, and the dog food bag. I picked up drive-thru on the way home from work. I let the answering machine take the weight of all of my calls. My husband became my caddy, as I instructed him to take the groceries out of the trunk, to scrub the bathtub, and to move the bed so that I could reach *Moby Dick*, dropped behind the headboard after another long night of waiting for Ishmael and Queequeg to board the whaling ship, The Pequod.

    I did what I could, but there was really no way to completely rest. Even when I was flat on my back, I could feel my bones pressing down into the mattress, repelling from my organs like two negative charges. The only possible way to truly rest would have been with the help of a mesh hammock, hooked onto the sides of the bed like the dangling cables of a helicopter, ready to lift me away from my life like a rescued whale.

~

    I was living backwards. The effort it took me to keep putting one foot in front of the other left me completely exhausted. I might as well have been surrounded by the ocean, my calves aching from the constant pull. Every object that I saw echoed my struggle to get through the day: I could hear the pain of the wood floors as they creaked under my feet, my cotton shirt clung and itched around my cold arms like a bad rash, even my shadow held me accountable for its quick shrinking in the afternoon.

I didn't know where to go, mentally or physically. My body tried to hold onto its previous patterns, but I didn't have a blueprint for this new experience. I clung onto my writing, trying to find a place with some sense of structure, a place where my familiar words could find their trusted metaphors:

First Trimester

The desert roses have not returned,
unlike the rest of the blooms,
broken under the wild grass and weeds
covering the front bed.
This year, a set of purple lips
opened instead,
growing inches overnight
between the tulip stems
and brittle forsythia.

Inside, everything moves
and is still.
The clock ticks,
the calendar gets crossed off,
breakfast becomes lunch
becomes dinner.
I take the wild bloom,
leave its long stem
smothered in the water
of a tall vase.

> *Within hours it has wilted,*
> *the wetness dripping off its petals,*
> *its soft pink center*
> *too drenched and tired*
> *to hold its weight any longer.*

There was no moving forward in this state. My only assurance was that another second would go by after that one had ended.

~

There were four limp fingers hanging out of me, four empty fingers of a latex glove the technician was using to improvise for a protective sleeve that was lost somewhere in the supply closet. I was back at the hospital, this time in the middle of the night, because there was no denying that something was definitely wrong. The blood was running out onto the towels under me while the nurse attempted to locate the pregnancy sac with the internal ultrasound probe.

She finally focused on a dark kidney shaped smear, and I swallowed as I saw a small motionless lump in the bottom of the sac. I knew what she was going to tell me, and she did. She said the word, *miscarriage*, and I realized that no one had actually spoken the word aloud since I had announced the pregnancy. Now I understood the weight of the word, how one slip of its first syllable had the power to kill, how one mention of the word could be a guarantee for its onset, for immediate jinxing and loss.

The tears came after my breath returned, and my husband curled his hands and head around my face and said he was sorry. I turned and looked, one last time, at the screen, at the tiny bits of matter that never became a baby.

The technician handed me a box of Kleenex. She said that there was a back exit that led directly to the parking lot. What she meant was that I was in no shape to walk back through the crowd of the injured and the diseased, waiting patiently for their own official diagnoses. I had already been evaluated, and there was nowhere left for me to go now, except out through the back door.

My hand found a pen and a napkin in the car, and I scribbled as we drove, aimlessly, around the Greater Baltimore Medical Center campus, until my doctor's office, located in the East Pavilion, opened at 9 a.m.:

Miscarriage

The embryo's shadow enlarges
across the screen,
one small lump
surrounded by
pulled strings of tissue.
I already know the answer,
have known since
the blood started,
since I began waking up nights
with an empty pit echoing
in my stomach.
"There should be a heartbeat by now,"
and I know the technician is trying to warn me,
to send the early flag down
before she passes the Kleenex
and tells me to get re-dressed.
I take one last look
at the shadow,
at the knot that could be
any random part of my body:
the pulled tendon of a finger,
a small cross section of the brain,
any part that doesn't move,
that never wakes up.

~

I tried to keep it together as the doctor motioned for my husband and me to sit down in the leather chairs across from his desk. It was 9:05 a.m. We had been awake since 2:30 a.m., since my husband had pulled our pickup into the ER parking lot, and we headed in for what I knew would only be bad news.

It turned out that I was officially having a "missed" miscarriage. The term sounded so easygoing, as if I had misplaced my pregnancy under the couch or down the heating vent. What it meant was that my miscarriage had not actually happened yet, as the unviable embryo had yet to expel itself from my body. It was still lodged inside of me like an old piece of food stuck above the garbage disposal. My body had become my worst enemy. First, it wouldn't accept the pregnancy, and now it wouldn't get rid of it.

The doctor told me that it could take days, or weeks, for the matter to expel from my body. He suggested that I should get a D & C, *a dilation and curettage*, to remove the miscarriage as soon as possible. It was the medical term for an abortion for the dead, for the removal of an unsuccessful pregnancy. I agreed. I couldn't continue to walk around for another day knowing that death had set up shop inside me. The doctor made a call from his desk and confirmed the D & C surgery for the afternoon. I watched him scribble D & C into his 2:30 slot with a light pencil.

"No eating or drinking before then because of the anesthesia," he said, as he closed his planner and pushed his chair back.

We followed his cue and stood up to leave. My husband held his hand forward to shake, like he had just made a big business deal with the doctor. I couldn't look at either of them. All I could think about was that I did not want this pregnancy to be *missed*. I wanted it to be *gone* and *erased*. I wanted to start over, with a clean slate and a body that was not tainted with a past attempt and failure.

~

I never realized that the mall was such a somber place: It was where you went after a bad break-up, when you needed an outfit for a funeral, or when you had a dead embryo inside you.

The floor on the high priced fourth level was shiny enough to reflect my discouraged face as we walked from shop to shop, my hands touching the merchandise without any connection to their actual functions. I needed to touch things, to be sure that I was still there, alive and breathing. The stores looked fake and blurry, like the first week after I had lasik eye surgery.

We had two hours before my D & C was scheduled. I didn't want to be home, and I didn't want to be at the hospital yet, which meant we had ended up there, at the mall, with my hand linked around my husband's arm. I wondered if the doctor knew how hard it was to keep moving until the afternoon, when there was a constant decaying reminder tight inside me.

A group of high school girls walked by, giggling and pointing ahead to a cute boy near the escalator. An elderly couple sat on one of the benches and shared a pretzel. I felt nauseated at the sight of their happiness. A young mother pushed a stroller by, yelling at her son, who was trying to climb out of the safety straps. I wanted to take the stroller and crack it over her head.

My husband used the pay phone in the food court to call my parents, and I could hear his voice quivering when he said, "She lost it." I stood next to the side of the pay phone while he spoke, looking at my face in the spotted metal reflection, the rusted spots covering my nose like growing cancers.

The food court began to fill with the lunch crowd, and I watched the lines start to thicken, the tables quickly covered with trays and paper cups. My mouth was completely dry from not eating or drinking for the last six hours, and my tongue felt chapped and cracked among the mucous that kept surfacing.

We started another aimless walk around the first level. The children's play area, Tiny Town, was packed, the toddlers climbing and falling over one another like little ants. I tried to keep from looking at them. It made me sick to my stomach to see the children playing, the mothers sitting on the side benches, coffee cups paused in their hands. It made me so sick that I felt like I could vomit up the pregnancy remains. *It would not be that bad*, I thought, *to have the miscarriage come out through my mouth, to let my tongue pull it forward from my gut like the slow tug of a fishing rod.*

~

We sat and waited in the obstetrics-admitting lounge, next to a set of great-grandparents-to-be counting the seconds until they could go back into the delivery area to meet their first great-grandchild. They snuggled on one of the couches, reminiscing about their own first child, born in a very different time, in the winter of 1934 on the floor of their living room. Their joy was so distanced from my emotional state that I couldn't understand the link between their smiles and the yellow balloons floating above their heads like portable suns. I was angry that they couldn't even tell that I had been pregnant. For all they knew, I was just someone else's sister, waiting to visit a newly arrived niece.

The nurse directed me into the back, through the double doors, and soon I was in a gray hospital gown, my belongings loose in a clear plastic bag, staring at an impressionistic yellow wildflowers painting on the wall. My doctor walked in, dressed in a pair of khakis and a denim shirt buttoned low enough that I could see a dark triangle of curly chest hair. He looked awkward without his white coat and stethoscope, like he was naked.

"The anesthesiologist will be coming in to talk to you soon," he said, and explained that the D & C should take about half an hour. He glanced over at my husband, who was fiddling with the metal screw on the side of his chair, and informed him that he was welcome to wait here while the surgery was performed.

After he left, I looked down at my feet, at the gray hospital slippers with elastic bunched just below my ankles. They were someone else's feet. They were the feet of an adult woman, a woman who was about to have surgery, an unwanted abortion, who had been pregnant for only a few fleeting seconds. It was not me, a little girl in warm slippers and a cotton gown, the girl who always picked the red lollipop at the bank, who liked to ride in the passenger side on the way home from church, who curled her toes back and forth at night to get to sleep.

~

Under. The first image that came to my mind was being buried alive. I could see my fingers scraping the wooden boards above me, clawing until splinters broke through my skin. I could barely hear my screams, so muffled under the earth that no one would even suspect it was anything but a slight wind whipping through a tree.

Here, in the hospital, *under* would mean erasing time. The drip of anesthesia would be my mother's hand, taking me home after a bad day at school. I would welcome the blackness, knowing that when I woke up the pregnancy would be gone; my body would be scraped clean like an empty batter bowl.

When I actually did wake up all I could focus on was the cramping, so strong that I swore I was going to wet the hospital bed. I started yelling that I had to go to the bathroom. In the background, I faintly heard a nurse telling my husband that I only thought I had to go. *What does she know?* I questioned. I wanted to show the nurse that I was right. I smiled as a warm wetness spread between my legs and I went back to sleep.

An hour later, after fully coming to, I declared that the bed needed to be changed. "No, it doesn't, sweetie," the same nurse replied, her voice clearer and louder than in my earlier memory. "You are fine. It just feels like you have to go."

She handed me a pamphlet titled *Miscarriage: Questions and Answers*, and left to get my discharge instructions. I opened it and tried to read the first question, but my vision was still so blurry that all I could make out were the words *devastating* and *unfair*. I folded it back into its even tri-fold and handed it to my husband. He stuffed it into my purse and helped me to get back into my clothes, my thighs still quivering from the pulse of the surgery.

My doctor came in and advised me to take a few days off from work, to rest as much as possible, and to wait a couple of months before trying again. His words sounded scripted.

"It's very common," he said. "You'll start hearing a lot of stories from other women about their miscarriages."

I felt anything but common. My anger boiled just below the surface, and I wished a miscarriage on him, some way for him to understand what I was feeling, to know his words were not helping me at all.

Back at home, I was beyond discouraged. I thought I would feel better after the surgery. Instead, I felt empty, like a failure, and every cramp reminded me that my plans had not worked. There would be no baby, only another two weeks of bleeding. I thought I would be back to the former self I remembered from before the pregnancy attempt. Now I knew that my old self was gone. I had to find a compromise for the mind and body that somehow still went by my old name.

Part Two

Halfway

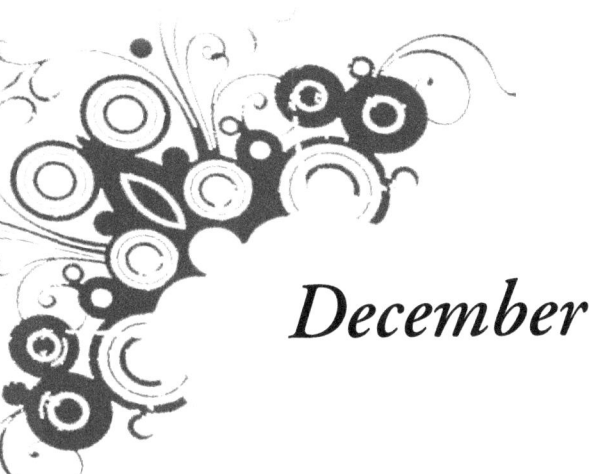

December

There was a large yellow card sitting in my office mailbox with faded pastel tulips and a rainbow on the cover. When I opened it up, I found an array of quotes penned by my coworkers, with phrases like *Tomorrow is a new day*, and *Life has its difficult times*.

I pictured my coworkers secretly passing the card around the day before, trying to think of something appropriate to write besides the customary *So Sorry For Your Loss*. How could they really understand the miscarriage? To them, it was not a real loss. A real loss had to begin to actually end. They never knew the beginning, while I had given myself over to the potential baby weeks ago, within seconds of reading the positive pregnancy test. They only knew I miscarried because I told them. To them, I might never have been pregnant at all.

There were not any greeting cards available to articulate this lack of shared experience. I made a mental note to start a new series of miscarriage cards. Instead of flowers, suns, and seashells, I would sketch black cats, bottles of vodka, and tornadoes on the covers. The messages on the inside would read, *Sorry, but at least you can drink now! You'll feel like hell for awhile!* or *Sure glad I'm not you!* The cards would give a paper cut when touched, just so the giver could feel a little taste of the pain.

My coworkers tiptoed around me. The pregnant women took their conversations behind closed doors. It felt like I had a disease, something fatal that made people uncomfortable to be around me. I realized that I was on *that end* of the conversation, the person people were whispering about:

"Do you think she's okay?" I heard the new girl ask as I walked by the lunchroom.

"My cousin had four miscarriages in a row," the receptionist whispered to my boss as I slipped into the shipping room to mail some invoices.

"It must be so hard," said one of the pregnant women, her hands cradling her tiny belly like a protective shield, "you know, with us here." She was in her office with the door almost closed, talking to the other pregnant woman.

"Did she do anything, you know, wrong?" I couldn't see the other woman, but I could hear her voice from behind the door.

"I did see her drinking a beer at the happy hour last month."

I gulped. I should have stormed in, just to make them stop talking about me, but my legs wouldn't move and my arms were dead weights at my sides. Finally, after a couple of minutes, I pried myself from the stone stance and walked into their office. The women had changed their topic to a debate about which hospital had the prettiest delivery room.

Their voices immediately stopped, and their hands suddenly became busy, rummaging through desk drawers for paper clips and addressing envelopes for next week's mailings. I was an outcast, with a capital M cut up and down my chest. I was there and not there, my body just off center from the rest of the ordinary, oiled up, and smoothly operating world.

~

My mother called in hysterics. My sister was gone again, this time without a note. I should have known. I should have pieced together her recent weight loss, the dark circles under her eyes, and the constant sniffles, but I had been so focused on my pregnancy and the miscarriage that she had slipped out of the sides of my peripheral vision.

We had been through this before, her junior year, the first time she ran away, leaving a note about her need to be with people who understood her. I went in search of her, physically that time, knocking on the boarded up buildings behind her high school, calling her friends and threatening them for her location. None of it helped. She had strolled back on her own, eventually, unaware of the sharp crack that she had caused in our lives, and reluctantly agreed to go into the adolescent outpatient program at Sheppard Pratt, the local psychiatric hospital. It was there that she really learned how to play the game, how to buy the drugs that covered the traces of the drugs and which bail bondsmen would show up the quickest. Deep down, I hadn't ever really believed that she wanted to get clean. She had just appeased my parents to bide some time.

This time I knew that nothing I did physically would matter. I didn't even consider chasing after her old shadow of a self. She was *under* now, and I had learned that no one could wake her up from her addiction but herself. The disease had come back to her like a familiar ex-lover. I worked on a poem, a letter that I wished I could mail, while I waited for my own bleeding to stop:

> *Sister,*
>
> *The police call every few days*
> *to see if we have heard from you.*
> *The same possibility*
> *each time the phone rings,*
>
> *that perhaps, one day,*
> *your tired voice will be there*
> *saying Come pick me up.*
> *I've had enough.*
>
> *How to live with this*
> *hole of un-control*
> *is something I cannot figure out.*
>
> *At first, it was only*
> *the lack of sleep,*
> *days without eating.*
>
> *Now, I'm trying to make myself forget,*
> *make the hours fly by*
> *simply for the sake of passing.*
>
> *Waking is hardest.*
> *Not recognizing your life*
> *only happens to other people.*
>
> *You are out there, high,*
> *sleeping with your dealer,*
> *wandering from street to street*
> *in search of a party,*
> *some happiness that is always*
> *just waiting to happen.*
>
> *Sister, I cannot get*
> *inside your head.*

*I cannot even start
to figure out the pieces
that must have broken
so many years ago.*

*At night I try to send
you a message through the air.
All I can think of
is a field of black poppies,
dim and old like a forgotten dream.*

*Where do I send this poem?
You have no address.
Where, when there is nowhere
for you to fit.*

*This is a poem about me,
Sister. It always was.
Can you see that?*

*I wait, and another day
goes by.*

*Sister, are you alive?
What can I write?
This is a poem about me.
Sister. A poem.*

Can't you see?

    I hated her for what she was continuing to do to herself and to our family. I hated that my mom couldn't look me in the eye without crying, and that my father was now cleaning his guns every time I was over. I hated myself for not recognizing what was right under my nose, for thinking my sister had to be like me, searching for the truth through words, instead of the unforgiving residue of powder and needles.

~

I could feel my anxiety returning. At first, it was moments of dizziness and shortened breath. Then I noticed that I kept waking up earlier and earlier, the alarm clock advertising its bright red numbers like the neon letters of an all night bar.

It was the same type of anxiety that I had experienced the year before, when my sister disappeared for the first time, and I was teaching at a girls' Catholic high school, my sister's drug habits tucked silently into the protection of my professional pockets. I didn't tell anyone at the school about my daily fear, that my mother would one day leave a message on my machine that would start with the dreaded, *I have some terrible news.* I sat through the faculty room lunches, listening to the other teachers blame parents for their failing students, sure that someone else at home had to be at fault for the girls' negative behaviors.

I looked out at my ninth grade class one afternoon and saw the girls' faces blurring back and forth like circus mirrors. I thought I was losing my mind. I thought I had a brain tumor or a rare form of cancer that was quickly taking hold. It took a month of appointments before I found a doctor who told me the truth: that it was all in my head. As soon as he said it, I broke down and did what I should have done months before. I wrote my resignation letter: *I regretfully write this resignation letter after much thought, feeling that my departure is the right thing to do at this time. I appreciate the learning experiences that I have had at your institution, but my gut tells me that it is time to move on, to travel down a new path in my life.* What I really meant to write was: *If I do not quit this job, I will have to be committed. You can take your holier than thou thoughts and kiss my ass!* I had my husband draw a pair of red lips on one of my butt cheeks the day that I dropped the resignation letter into the principal's mailbox.

~

The only person I knew who had been actually committed was my uncle, my mother's brother. He had been living at Springfield State Hospital in Carroll County since I was six years old. That was the last time I saw him at my grandparents' house, running up the basement steps with smoke billowing from his head. I could still see his body rolling uncontrollably like a wild animal on the front lawn while my grandfather smothered the flames with a gray blanket. My grandparents committed him that year, in 1976, when he started setting blazes in the basement and painted all of the furniture in the house red.

One of the first poems that I ever wrote was about him, an exercise from my high school creative writing instructor, to describe a vivid memory from your past:

1975

Back when my uncle had not yet
been pulled by his long red braid
into the state institution,
I would take walks with him
behind my grandparents' house in DC.

He would lead me past the sewer tunnels
gripped by graffiti,
and have me spell out the cuss words,
the letters fresh in my mind
from my recent spelling lessons.

*His tattooed arms blurred the sight
of the Mexican men
huddled by the iron grated gate,
their thin sweaty fingers
passing a pipe between them.*

*That was when the smell of marijuana
was only sweet smoke to me
and the beer cans and glass
floating down the stream
were prisms and special treasures.*

*At the end of our walks he would point
to a caged sewer pipe and describe
the lion who lived in there,
hungry, and just waiting
for some little children to eat.*

*Between laughing and crying,
I would scale the metal bars,
hurrying through the long seconds,
feeling the lion's breath
heavy on my heels.*

*This flame-haired man frightened
and fascinated me
with his long pointed nails,
cut-off sleeveless shirts,
and album covers full
of sad, naked Asian women.*

*The dark red of his face,
his red room in the basement,
even the way he drank his milk
was the same redness
of my forgotten dreams.*

*It was the same red smell
of the magic store down the street
and I wondered how he could live
in the aftermath of red dreams
and the smell of true red magic
and stay sane.*

I went to see my uncle at the state hospital a couple of times with my mother when I was in college. His skin cancer had progressed so much by then that it looked like a bird had pecked out entire pieces of his face. He never spoke to me during those visits. I was not sure if he even remembered me, a scared six-year-old girl from his previous life. He just took the stale bread that my mother always brought at his request, broke it up into small pieces with his dirty fingers, and threw it up in the air for the sea gulls to catch. They circled him, and from far away, someone could have mistaken him for their trainer. I could tell then that he had passed the point of connection with any other human. The birds were his sole companions. He did not need words for them to understand him. He did not need laws or rules to stay in their graces.

~

I was back in the therapist's office, trying to articulate the pain of my miscarriage, but all that kept coming out of my mouth were stories about my sister. I took up the full hour complaining about my sister's lack of respect, of the years I had spent picking her up from parking lots, wanting to believe the excuses: she had a cold, she hated to eat, and she was chronically late because she always forgot to wear her watch.

I gave the therapist a copy of one of my latest poems, entitled "Death," a not so subtle poem symbolizing my current state of mind:

Death

Moves across the room
like a silent serpent,
eyeing each ignorant body
in between the quick reflexes

*of his gray scales,
our names covering
the pores of his slick body.*

*Everyone keeps talking,
watching football,
eating their dinner.*

*Look, I want to scream,
he's here, under the couch
with his fangs wide open,
on the top of the ceiling fan,
waiting for the next spin.*

*Everyone is oblivious.
They are too intent
on the taste of Cheese Whiz
with their Wheat Thins.*

*I look down at my plate
and move a few lettuce leaves
around in the dressing.
The dressing is gray, too,
with little pebbles
and flakes of old paint.*

*I want to spread
the liquid onto my skin,
to build up an armor
stronger than any metal.
But, instead,
I sit quietly and listen,
and, like usual,
no one notices the difference.*

The therapist scanned the poem, nodded, and then stuffed it into the back of my folder while she whispered, "We don't want to call attention to this one." I immediately pictured the director of the therapy office leafing through my file in the middle of the night, flashlight in hand, perusing each page of notes until he reached "Death," tucked neatly in the back. I could see the flashlight dropping, the light cracking across the ceiling, as he reached for the phone to call the powers at be to have me committed, pulled straight out of my bed and into a straight jacket.

I mentioned to the therapist that my mother had been going to Nar-Anon, and that it seemed to be helping her to deal with my sister's problems. The therapist suggested that I should go to the next meeting. Our hour passed in what seemed like a few minutes, and I made another appointment for the next week. The day before my scheduled appointment, the therapist called to say she had to cancel due to a family emergency. I decided not to call her back. I couldn't stomach the thought of rescheduling my feelings.

~

My mother stood up and read the first step out of her little blue book: "We admitted that we were powerless over *our addict*, and that our lives had become unmanageable." I was at her Nar-Anon meeting, held in one of the rooms at Sheppard Pratt, the same wing where my sister had once attended her outpatient drug program. It immediately reminded me of the Fast and Testimony meetings of my childhood at the Mormon Church, the long hours of faith testimonies, tears, and endless tissues climbing out of my mother's purse. I always begged my mother not to go up to the podium and stand up in front of all those people in the congregation, leaving my sister and me alone on the pew. I didn't want her opening up our family's secrets like a can of sardines, exposing every gill and delicate bone. I sat waiting for the words that might come out of her mouth at any moment: *My daughter wet her pants behind the shed last week*, or *My daughter picked her nose this morning before she came down to breakfast*. It was always a relief when she sat back down at the pew after a couple of minutes of thanking God and the church for her blessings. My life was only secure with her next to me, her body heat comforting me, letting me know that everything would be okay.

At this Nar-Anon testimony meeting she was not thanking anyone, but explaining that she did not recognize the signs of my sister's recent relapse. She was in denial, hopeful that my sister would never go back to her old habits, and naïve in thinking her love could stop its return. Now that my sister was gone, my mother could only linger, barely breathing without any children moving around in the house and aging walls that advertised her worst fears.

After my mother sat back down into her chair, the man sitting on the other side of her quickly stood up and covered his face with his hands as he started to cry. I watched my mother instinctively place her hand on his elbow. While the man gasped and the rest of the room was uncomfortably silent, I thumbed through the light blue Nar-Anon booklet on the seat next to me. Towards the back of the booklet, I found

Signs of Addiction:

1. *Deterioration of physical health and appearance*
2. *Increase in sleep and/or exhaustion*
3. *Neglect of school, work, or other responsibilities*
4. *Irrational crying and/or rage*

5. *Emotional numbness*
6. *Frequent secretive behavior*
7. *Decrease in appetite*
8. *Increase in accidents and carelessness*
9. *Withdrawal from family, friends, and intimate relationships*
10. *Onset of anxiety, depression, confusion, and/or psychosis*

It was like reading a definition of my sister, and maybe myself as well.

"It's my son," the man finally spit out when he was composed enough to talk. I took my eyes off the booklet and watched the wrinkles in his face continue to pucker like a prune.

"He's been given 5-10 years. I think I'm losing my marriage from it." He brought his hands back to his face. My mother continued to hold his elbow, like an awkward sling. I did not feel secure or safe at this meeting, even knowing that my mother had stepped down from the podium without giving away any of my secrets. I finally saw the testimony room for what it really was: a group of adults trying to understand, to make some sense of the insanity that life had thrown at them. This time, there was no one to give me comfort, to make me feel like everything would be okay. This time I was one of them, looking for light in the dark.

At the end of the meeting the group gathered into a circle, and I felt my mother gently squeeze my hand as the room of voices repeated: *God, grant me the serenity to accept the things I cannot change, the courage to change the things I can, and the wisdom to know the difference.*

~

I examined my palm for my dissection point, any scar or fold in my lifeline that might represent this miscarriage and point of tragedy in my life. One of my former students from the Catholic high school taught me about dissection points. She was a twelfth grader whose father had died the year before I came to the school. She showed me her own point of crossing, a tiny groove in the bottom of her palm. She explained to me that her dissection point came earlier than it did for most people, and that most would not come across their own points until later on in their lives.

I could not help but wonder if she had created this perspective herself, or if her mother had explained it to her, in the late night hours of a depressing night, as their hands met above her mother's now half-empty bed. It made the other girls in the class seem so young and ignorant, as they traded yearbooks and passed notes when I wasn't looking.

They don't know what's coming, I remember thinking, as I confiscated yet another bottle of bright red nail polish during seventh period. *They haven't met their points yet. Their worlds are still safe. Events are still within their control. It is just a matter of time before all of that will change.*

There. I thought I saw it: a small wrinkle a third of the way up my lifeline. If I stretched my palm open it disappeared, but then it returned when I relaxed my hand. It was like any addiction; it came back when no one was looking.

~

"I have some terrible news," the message began on the answering machine, my mother's voice dark and low like a grave. It was the message that I had feared for the past two years. My heart dropped into my feet, imagining my sister's body cold and stiffened on the dirty floor of a rented motel room, her user friends long gone, replaced with rats and cockroaches. I swallowed as the walls of the room started to close in around me.

"Your uncle has terminal cancer," she continued, and the walls suddenly wavered and began to slowly move back to their positions around me. "They've given him nine months to live. His skin cancer has spread into his entire body."

I was relieved, in a very selfish way, that it wasn't my sister who was dying, but a relative who was more like a stranger, a name in a newspaper, made out of ink and paper instead of flesh and blood.

My mother seemed to handle the news of his impending death pretty well. She didn't seem surprised, like she had been waiting for this day, after years of visiting him at the hospital and watching the skin cancers eat away his face. She started going through her photo albums, looking for a picture of him when he was younger. She wanted to find a picture that showed him before the mental illness began, proof to everyone that he had been normal once, in a time long before anyone could remember. She wanted to find a picture of *before*, of the freckle on his cheek that she used to think looked like a treasure spot X when they were growing up, or of the front tooth that she remembered dangled for weeks from his gum, not at all anxious to release itself from his seven year old smile.

~

Instead of waiting two months to try again, like the doctor suggested, I decided to wait two weeks. I was like a sneaky teenager, pretending to accept my two month grounding term while I secretly planned to climb out of my window that night to meet a boyfriend down the street at the graveyard.

My plans were organized and ready. On Monday, I jumped into bed naked and freshly shaven, a guarantee for some action. On Tuesday, I dug out the cherry flavored love potion from our honeymoon. I called my husband at work on Wednesday and told him that I wasn't wearing any underwear. On Thursday, I accidentally left *When Mary met Sally* in the DVD player. It did the trick. We were exhausted by Friday, our bodies settling back into the usual indentations on either side of the bed.

Having sex again made me feel like I was back in control of my life. I was an adult now, not a child or a healing consequence. I didn't care what the doctor had instructed. He already had one big strike against him. He should have known how to prevent the miscarriage. He should have understood. I was in charge now, and my life waited to be served on a *Victoria's Secret* platter.

~

I had only been on the Peter Pan bus for half an hour, and already I knew the weekend would not be the release that I hoped it would be. I was on the same route to New York that I had traveled at least twenty times since college. It was the same smell of stale fabric from the seat in front of me, the same man singing from beneath his headphones three rows behind me, and the same slow driver taking another puff of his cigarette before climbing back on board the bus. However, this time there was no anticipation of what might happen in the city, of what handsome man might stumble across my path, or which wealthy patron might see my poetic potential from just watching me walk down the street, offering me a studio and a generous stipend for my inevitable talent.

Bad Boys, starring Martin Lawrence and Will Smith, came onto all of the small televisions which were hanging from four locations inside the bus. None of the jokes were funny, though the man to my left kept laughing hysterically. I tried to read *Moby Dick*, which I had brought along in my backpack, but the bus kept braking, and I had to stop due to the headache which quickly surfaced. It was a rather lengthy chapter, listing the types of whales and cataloguing the origins of each of their sightings. It was too much information for me to digest, and it was all I could do just to hold my breath as we inched through the Lincoln Tunnel, swallowed completely within the aging concrete below the Hudson.

My heart felt like it was going to break through my chest by the time I got to the tenth flight of stairs of my friend's Brooklyn apartment building. She was waiting at the top of the steps in her fuzzy slippers, ready for our usual stimulating conversations about men and the arts. I wanted to tell her that everything was different now, that I couldn't smile anymore or put on mascara with any amount of conviction. Instead, I hugged her and told her that it was wonderful to see her and that the bus ride was fine.

She did her best to entertain me. We went to the Guggenheim and a tasty French restaurant where I ordered roast duckling with orange sauce and a cabernet. My mood didn't change, though. Even the wine didn't do its usual trick—I just felt more tired, dazed, and dizzy. Two days later and $200 poorer, I took the same dusty bus back to the Baltimore Travel Plaza. This time Jackie Chan fought his way through our route down Interstate 95. *I had a great time,* I emailed back to my friend after returning home. It would have been great in my former life, before the miscarriage, when friends, art, good food, and wine were just that.

~

I made a conscious effort to become distracted with the upcoming Christmas holiday. I wanted to pretend that I was thinking about something else besides the lost baby. I started with decorations. Due to my lack of funds, the dollar store was my only option, so I stocked up on red bows, fake garland, molded ornaments and red vinyl tablecloths. Even the dogs got stockings, cheap knit socks that said, *"Dogs Love Christmas Too!"* and *"Doggie's been a Good Boy!"* I bought and played the Charlotte Church Christmas CD, *Dream a Dream,* non-stop from morning until night.

I made all of my friends and family homemade oil and vinegar jars and added chili peppers, basil, and rosemary to spice up the flavors. I carefully matched each person's personality with one of the particular spices. My mother got a lone twig of rosemary floating in a layer of olive oil. Two sturdy basil leaves stuck together in the vinegar layer of my father's batch. I even made one for my sister, in case she re-surfaced before the holiday, combining one of each spice and then stirring them until the mixture looked like a confused salad dressing. The chili peppers clung to the sides of the jar while the basil and rosemary tangled at the bottom of the liquid. I pretended it was a magic potion strong enough to bring my sister home, a jar as precious as frankincense or myrrh.

Marshall's discount store had a gaudy sweater on sale with bright sequins sewn into a green wreath on its front and a pair of matching socks fastened to its collar. It looked quite fitting among the icicle lights that I ordered my husband to hang from every mildewed gutter around the house. Mistletoe swung in the dining room, suspended from a string tied to our rotating ceiling fan.

I set up the nativity that had been buried in the attic for the last three years and looked at the warm straw coming out of the manger while I rubbed my finger across the baby's smooth head. Mary seemed to flinch at the presence of my knuckle, nervous at my hand being so close to her child. I moved the pointy pieces of straw away from his body so that she would know I didn't wish him any harm.

The Christmas distraction worked. I was lucky. I could have picked chocolate, speeding, or heroin. It could just as easily have been piercings or tattoos.

~

I reluctantly made myself pull over into the Rite Aid parking lot on my way to the high school choir kick-off. I counted the days since the

D & C in my head: 38. 38 days, and I still hadn't gotten my period. There was a special on the end display of the fourth aisle: two for one generic brand pregnancy tests for $9.99. I snatched them up, along with five boxes of Christmas cards that caught my eye at the register. The cards had a sketch of the nativity printed in black ink on the front. The baby Jesus' head centered each drawing with a glowing yellow halo, the only color on the page. When the clerk scanned the cards through the register, I could hardly believe that I was buying them. I never bought religious cards. Nevertheless, I couldn't leave the baby Jesus on the cold metal shelf. I couldn't leave the halo muted by the fluorescent lights that ran the entire length of the store, artificial and grungy like worn lanes at a bowling alley.

After all of my purchases were in the bag, I walked over to the McDonald's across the parking lot. The sweat started to drip across my forehead as I waited in the second stall of the bathroom. The blank box slowly dampened, and I watched, staring at it for over three minutes. *Nothing.* There was only a blank wet square next to the example square. *Nothing.* Only the sample line was glowing: a proud pre-dyed line advertising its impossible perfection like a new pink bikini.

I threw the test into the trashcan, stuffed the extra test into my purse, and got to the fundraising kick-off five minutes late. The choir director didn't even notice, since she was in the midst of reprimanding the sopranos for not practicing over the weekend. When I finally returned to the office, I immediately started working on my Christmas cards. I wrote the summary in third person on the inside of the cards: *Kathy had a miscarriage. She hates life and only talks to other people when necessary. Her sister is missing. Her uncle is dying. She is thinking about taking up Scotch as a hobby after the holidays. She hopes you have a Merry Christmas!*

~

One good thing about not being pregnant was that I could drink heavily again, which was the main reason I was looking forward to the engagement party of a former English department colleague from the Catholic high school, held a few days before Christmas at Mick O' Shea's Irish Pub. The thoughts of dark Guinness floated through my head as the night approached, the black stout sliding down my throat like thick syrup, foam left across my upper lip in a scruffy mustache.

Before we left, I decided to take the second pregnancy test, more as an *It's okay to get sloshed* confirmation, since my period had still not arrived. I fished it out of my purse, peeled the wrapper off, and peed on the stick. The wetness quickly darkened the empty square and there, faintly, appeared a little pink line, so light that it might have been a shadow or an eyelash. This time I didn't need the rest of the two minutes that it recommended waiting to know I had been given another chance. My eyes welled up, and I had to tell my husband three times that everything was fine as I splashed water over my face and applied an extra thick layer of eyeliner. I didn't want to tell him yet. I didn't want to jinx this pregnancy. I didn't want to tell anyone. I didn't want anything to be the same about this pregnancy. I took a big breath and held my knowledge tight in the pit of my stomach.

No one even noticed that I didn't drink at the engagement party.

They were too busy being sympathetic about my miscarriage, telling me repeatedly that they were sorry, and that I was sure to get pregnant again *one day.*

~

I could feel the letters P-R-E-G-N-A-N-T starting to push out across my forehead as soon as we walked into my grandparents' house on Christmas morning. I was burning to tell someone. My cheeks were flushed, and my stomach already felt tight against my pants' zipper.

The relatives had uncomfortable looks on their faces, the kind that people have when someone in the room has recently experienced a loss. I noticed the way my aunt took my coat directly off my shoulders and how my grandmother left her hand on my arm longer than usual. Everyone was caring, but no one actually talked about the recent tragedies of my miscarriage, my missing sister, and my dying uncle. They talked about the snow and the price of gas. The house felt stagnant to me. People were talking and moving, but there was nothing holding everyone's actions together. The air was splintered, and I wondered if the rest of my life would be like this. I quietly unzipped my pants underneath my big red sweater while my grandfather said the blessing for the meal.

After breakfast, we opened gifts for over an hour. My mother kept a pile for my sister in the back corner of the room. We pretended that we didn't see them there, pushed out of the way like a punished child.

I carefully peeled the tape away from my own presents, knowing that my fingers had to be exposing my secret. The middle of the living room quickly filled with wrinkled wrapping paper and torn boxes, and I left the room to get a few trash bags from the kitchen, desperate to escape all of the mouths that kept talking and sucking in the air.

I tried to keep from crying as I hunted for the trash bags under the sink. The household chemicals mocked me with their poisonous colors, deep blues that looked tasty enough to drink and warm yellows that were the shade of lemons and hay. I wondered who decided to dress death in such appealing colors. They were the colors that a child would want to explore, the colors of crystal ponds and magical fountains.

I spotted the trash bags behind the Drano and took a big breath before returning to the inevitable *after* Christmas in the living room, the remnants of another year unwrapped, and like usual, never as glorious as anticipated.

~

Please, no. I wiped again, and found another blood spot next to the first mark. It was the day after Christmas, and I was the only one at work besides my boss. I dropped the toilet paper into the bowl and flushed, watching the stained toilet paper disappear down the drain into the world of decaying pipes and bacteria eating creatures.

I tried calling my husband at work six times, but he was either pulling a motor or test-driving a car. My boss kept making inappropriate Christmas and Hanukkah jokes. I pretended to laugh, watching my fingers trace the numbers on the pads of the telephone. The second hand of the clock ticked on the wall, its slow rotations pulling me forward with sluggish speed.

After I got home, I paced the floor, walking back and forth between the rooms until I started to get dizzy. My husband finally pulled into the driveway. The second that he walked through the door, I started crying and spilled the news about the pregnancy and the spotting. I could see the shock in his face, his eyes forced open in surprise.

"Already?" he repeated. "You're pregnant already? You're sure?"

"Yes, I'm sure, but I don't want to tell anyone," I pleaded.

"You don't have to," he reassured me, "You don't have to." However, it was too late to hold in my fear, the floodgates had opened, and I drenched his shirt for the rest of the night.

~

I was obsessed with the spotting, going to the bathroom every fifteen minutes to see if there was more blood. I could barely remember a time when going to the bathroom was not stressful, when it was not a reminder of my past failure, of a glimpse of my forthcoming tragedy. I couldn't think about anything but blood. It was everywhere that I looked—behind the cut on my knee from the old razor, between the meat and the dried bone of the chicken drumstick I forced down for dinner, even in the red-veined eyes of my basset hound as he looked up and begged for some attention.

My husband was oblivious to my obsession. He only understood the spotting as a small factor of my pregnancy. He didn't see that it transcended the bathroom and the toilet paper. It wasn't just a symptom, like hemorrhoids or pimples. It carried my entire body and mind through every moment of the day. It was like a fever I couldn't shake.

Could there actually be a husband or boyfriend out there who was just as obsessed as I was, who went through his wife's dirty clothes hamper, looking for traces of blood on her panties? Was there ever a man who had woken in a sweat, his heart racing from another reoccurring nightmare about stained sheets?

~

I woke my husband on New Year's Eve morning and paged the doctor on call from the phone in the kitchen. I tried to keep my feet within the boundaries of the white laminate squares while I waited for the doctor to return my page. The bleeding was worse. After ten minutes, the phone rang in my hand, and I was actually startled, the ring confirming that I had set forces outside of my home into action. The tired voice of a woman with a Mid-Eastern accent met my ear. I told her about my current bleeding and my past miscarriage. She suggested that I should go to the emergency room, just in case it was another miscarriage.

I called my mother and immediately started crying when she answered the phone. She, too, was completely surprised that I was even pregnant again. She agreed to meet me at the hospital, and I piled more pads into my purse as we headed out the door, reciting my upcoming diagnosis of infertility in my head.

We found the last spot on the roof level of the parking garage and made our way to the lobby, where my mother was already waiting. Her hair was sticking straight up in the back like a frightened bird. I tried to pat it down for her as we hugged, and she told me that everything would be okay.

The emergency room was packed, and I had to wait over an hour before the nurse called me into the back. She hooked me up to the blood pressure machine and asked me the date of my last period, which I had to explain to her three times, was actually three months earlier because of the miscarriage and the D & C. I changed into the hospital gown with the familiar gray hue and scrawny ties and waited in the examining room. The doctor, a young man with a buzz cut, strolled in close to forty minutes later.

He asked me about my symptoms and pressed down on my stomach with his warm hands. He told me that I could possibly have some of the previous pregnancy still in me, which would cause a positive pregnancy test and a heavy period. He left to order the blood work, and I imagined a scrap of dead baby inside me, stuck like an old fly on a sticky strip. Could I have fabricated this second pregnancy? Was it possible that my hormones had allowed me to believe in this conception while the missed bit of embryo continued to shrivel inside?

My mother passed the time by telling me a story about a woman she knew who had a D & C for pre-menopausal excessive bleeding without knowing she was actually pregnant. The fetus survived the D & C and the daughter who was born from that pregnancy got to go on to tell the story that she was so strong she even survived a D & C. I tried to smile, but I kept biting the insides of my cheeks with my teeth.

A nurse came in to take my blood, and another half hour passed. I counted all of the gray stitches around the seam of my gown: 175 of them. I started to re-count just the stitches that were facing east when the doctor parted the curtain, stepped in, and announced that I was indeed pregnant, and almost six weeks along!

"Six? How could she already be six weeks along?" my mother gasped.

My husband smiled.

"Well, she is," the doctor said, "I'm going to request an ultrasound. They can do it upstairs." He started to leave to find a prescription pad for my ultrasound referral then suddenly turned around. "Do you want this baby?" he asked, startling me with the question.

"Yeh," I replied, caught off guard with the idea that I wouldn't.

"Good," he sighed and parted the curtain.

Six weeks. Six weeks was a long time. Six weeks was the time it took me to go through my prenatal vitamin pack. Six weeks was how long I had to wait to change my first set of pierced earrings. Six weeks was the life span of a mosquito, of two high school boyfriends, of my first late period in college. Six weeks was an eternity.

We waited another twenty minutes before a man came by with a gurney, ready to wheel me upstairs to the on-site radiology department. I felt like the gurney treatment was a little unnecessary, but he quickly snapped that he was just following orders, and I climbed onto the moveable bed. He was a huge man, so wide that he couldn't judge corners, and we hit at least four walls with the left wheel of the gurney.

A pale pixy haired technician came out from behind the double doors of the radiology department and helped to fit the gurney through the door. She gave the man the evil eye, so I knew there had to be more to his hazardous pushing than I would ever know. My mother and husband waited outside the cramped room while the technician did the usual routine: squirting cold jelly across my stomach, and then rubbing the transducer across my skin. I watched the screen with apprehension—hoping for a tiny bleep, some sign that this was different from the last pregnancy. She kept moving the transducer back and forth, too fast to be a sign that she has found anything concrete yet. She finally packed up the external ultrasound and said she would have to do an internal ultrasound since it was so early in the pregnancy.

I was relieved to climb off of the gurney and pee, to empty my uncomfortably full bladder before the next procedure began. She instructed me to insert the internal probe, and then took control of it before she began moving it around. Here I was again, having a nurse fish for clues inside of me with a piece of hard plastic. I asked her what she was seeing as she measured and clicked, entering numbers into the keyboard beneath the screen like a secret code.

"This is the pregnancy sac," she said, pointing to the dark oval running down the middle of the screen. She clicked around a small dark spot in the middle. "And this is the start of a pregnancy." She measured and clicked, then measured and clicked some more. "It's so early, though, I can't be quite sure if there is a heartbeat—I might have seen one, but I'm not exactly sure- I can't write it down because I'm not positive."

"Does this look like a miscarriage to you?" I asked her, my lips quivering.

She turned to me then and looked directly into my eyes. "I don't think so," she paused, "But it's still early."

I wanted to hug her, to thank her for being the first person to give me a tiny bit of hope. I wondered if she had ever miscarried, if she had been in the same position, knees up to her shoulders, while another technician searched her body for any sign of a baby.

"Call your doctor," she recommended. "He'll probably advise getting a follow up ultrasound in a couple of weeks." She was my angel, my first barer of good news.

"Do you want this baby?" she asked, repeating the same question that the doctor had previously asked me.

"Yes," I immediately responded, realizing she and the doctor must have heard "No" from enough women that it had become a standard question.

"Yes," I repeated, "I want this baby very much."

I left the hospital famished. I hadn't eaten since the night before, and I felt like I could eat a house. We stopped by Café Zen on the way home for sushi. I ordered the pregnancy safe versions: California Roll, Shrimp Roll, and Chesapeake Roll, moist bites of water, plant, and animal. The food tasted better than anything I had ever tasted before.

That night I was prepared for my New Year's celebration: a bottle of non-alcoholic sparkling grape juice, two wine glasses, the TV channel set for Dick Clark, salt and vinegar potato chips, and my pregnancy still intact inside me. By 10:30 p.m. I didn't think my eyelids would be able to stay open until midnight.

I didn't recognize any of the teenage musicians on *Dick Clark's New*

Year's Eve Rockin' Countdown. They all looked alike with their angst expressions and tight, dark jeans. I was so tired, but I still needed to get the fake wine out of the refrigerator. I closed my eyes for a minute. Just for a minute, I let myself believe that the world and my body did not need my attention. Just for a minute, I closed my eyes.

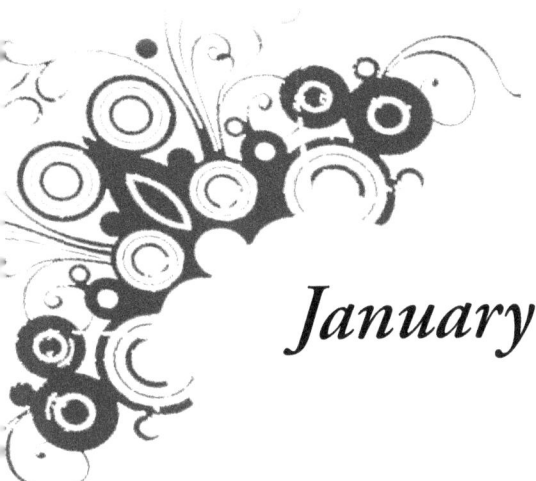

January

"Oh God, not now," I said aloud. The piece of toilet tissue was soaked with blood, lighter in color and thicker than the usual spotting that I had been having.

It was 9:05 a.m., and I was at work. I panicked, not knowing what to do. I had to tell someone. I pulled up my pants and ran into the nearest office, which happened to belong to the pregnant coworkers, and burst in with the news: "I think I'm having another miscarriage!" There were at least six women huddled around the coworkers' desks. Apparently, I had walked in on an early morning gossip session. The women looked at me like I had two heads.

"I'm pregnant again," I stuttered, suddenly remembering that I hadn't told anyone at work yet about the new pregnancy. My coworkers just stood there with their mouths open. I felt completely helpless and started crying.

Finally, one of the pregnant coworkers piped in, "Why don't we give you some privacy while you call your doctor." She helped to clear everyone from the room, and suddenly she was transformed into my mother: her nice designer linen suit covered with a red apron, her hands still warm from recent oven mitts. She even took on my mother's smell—a mix of pine tree, soap, and Christmas cookie. I needed her to be my mother, to tell me what I had to do, to make me understand there was logic in the direction that I was choosing, that an answer was waiting just because she said it was so.

I called my doctor and spoke to the nurse. "The bleeding is worse," I stuttered.

"Oh, hon, why don't you come in," she suggested.

"O.K.," I agreed and hung up. Now I had to tell my manager about the situation, who had to be suspecting something was up since every employee in the office was in a whispering huddle in the reception area.

I walked right into his office, looked him straight in the eye, and said, "I am pregnant and bleeding and need to go to the doctor's office." He just nodded and put his head down on his desk, a half eaten bag of M & M's and "Weekly Goals Left to Achieve" form directly under his forehead.

One of the elementary school reps volunteered to drive me to the doctor's office. The community group rep chimed in that she wanted to come along, too, for support. The elementary rep's concern seemed genuine. I suspected the community group rep saw an acceptable excuse for getting out of work.

I didn't even flinch as I dropped my clothes and draped the paper towel gown around my shivering body. Within a few seconds, the doctor had grabbed the lubricant and a cold speculum. The nurse rubbed my arm as he examined me, and I explained that the bleeding was heavier and pointed to my underwear resting on the chair, evidence that I wasn't making up this drama.

"Yep, there was some bleeding," the doctor said, scooting away from the table and snapping off his gloves. "But it looks like it has stopped now." How could he tell it had stopped? Did he know if the bleeding would start again?

"I'll send you for another ultrasound," he said nonchalantly, as if he was sending me in for an eyebrow wax. "Okay. Get dressed and I'll see you in my office."

I felt like a pupil, summoned to the principal's office. His dark wood desk and cabinet glared back at me with suspicion. All that was missing was the paddle for misbehavior. He finished scribbling notes in my file— *some bleeding, cervix closed*--as I squirmed in the chair on the other side of his desk.

"I didn't think it would happen again this soon," I blurted out, my body consciously clothed and warm after my recent exam. I waited for the lecture, for the *you deserve a miscarriage for getting pregnant again when I told you not to*.

"It must be meant to be," he smiled.

His response surprised me, and I didn't know what to say.

"I have scheduled an ultrasound for 1:00 at St. Joseph's—for your peace of mind—but I think you'll be okay," he stated.

Okay? Was it possible that everything would be okay? Or, was he just humoring me? With the constant bleeding, I couldn't imagine that anything could be all right. I wanted him to be able to see inside my body, to understand my blueprint, to know every blood vessel flowing through my uterus. I was frustrated that he couldn't, and that he had to send me to another place to find out if the pregnancy was still viable.

I grabbed my purse and walked out into the waiting area to tell my coworkers, who were both sitting there reading the latest *Baltimore: Top 100 Eats* magazine.

"I have an appointment at 1:00 at St. Joseph's," I announced to them. "Do you want to come?"

"Sure," blurted the elementary school rep.

"Definitely," said the community group rep. "Let's go get some lunch at the mall first. I want to run into Banana Republic while we're there."

We strolled around the mall for two hours before the elementary school rep decided to call our manager to update him on the situation. I could picture him downing five Tylenol with his morning snack of M & M's and Coke, extensively revising his projected sales goals for the day. I looked around at all of the people at the freshly wiped Food Court tables who were eating and talking without any care of the upcoming afternoon events, unaware of the blood rushing through their veins or the strong and even beats of their hearts. We stayed away from the first level, as I couldn't deal with seeing the children's play area, *Tiny Town,* and its shoe rack filled with little red boots and candy colored tennis shoes. The community group rep bought two outfits at Banana Republic and one at Anne Taylor.

I wasn't sure if the words would come out of my mouth when we finally arrived at St. Joseph's Hospital, and I asked the eighty-year-old nun on front desk duty where the radiology room was located. She looked down in slight disapproval at us, like we were asking to borrow pencils because we had accidentally broken ours, and directed us to the third floor. I imagined the nun at night, changing into her floor length white nightgown with the petite ruffle around the wrists and neck, feeling so proud that she had kept her body pure and untouched by any man. I wondered if she thought of herself as God's pinkie finger, a skinny bone that rose and fell with his direction. Did she view her reproductive organs, sagging breasts and wrinkly vagina as unnecessary components of her earthly body? Did she think they could disappear if she wished it hard enough?

We rode up the elevator, and my stomach churned as the weight of the elevator lifted for a brief moment before settling down onto the third floor.

"Can we watch them do the ultrasound?" the community group rep asked, like an anxious toddler as the elevator door slid open.

We finally found the radiology department at the end of the long hall. The receptionist gave me a bizarre look when I checked in and asked if my coworkers could come in to observe the ultrasound exam.

"Uh, sure," she said, obviously caught off guard with the unusual request. A technician came out into the waiting room and called my name. She looked like a rebellious Catholic school girl with her plaid mini-skirt and skimpy halter-top peeking out from beneath her white lab coat. I wondered how the nun downstairs felt about her attire, and I remembered the dirty looks that I used to get at the Catholic high school when I, as a teacher, arrived in my knee-high black leather boots.

We shuffled into the crowded white room, and the technician closed the door behind us before instructing me to do the usual: *Undress and have a seat up on the table.* She tried the external ultrasound on my stomach first, pushing the gelled transducer back and forth across my belly. My coworkers stared at the static bleeps that moved like slippery balloons across the monitor. Soon enough, she gave up and pulled out the internal probe for me to insert.

I suddenly knew exactly what my mother had meant when I had asked her, at eight years old, how she could possibly have given birth in front of the doctor and my father. The thought of anyone looking at my naked body then had felt equal to the amputation of an arm or leg. I imagined the violation to feel just as violent. She smiled and said, "When you love someone enough you will do anything."

And here I was, without a grain of modesty, spread eagle with a big plastic probe stuck up me in front of my coworkers. The technician looked down at the light blood trail that was beginning to stain the protective white paper underneath me. I clenched my teeth as she took the probe from me, and pushed it to the left and then twisted it to the right. A long dark sac appeared on the monitor, shaped like a kidney bean. There was a small wad in the center of the sac that resembled an old piece of chewing gum.

I blinked. It blinked. I blinked. It blinked again.

"There's a heartbeat," she said, and my coworkers rushed to the monitor, their eyebrows raised in such a way that I knew they had no clue what they were looking at on the screen. Nevertheless, I had seen it—a tiny speck blinking in and out like a weak firefly. I closed my eyes and re-opened them, just to make sure. It continued to blink.

This is real. This is real. This is real, I repeated to myself.

~

Waiting was the weight of my world. I felt completely isolated as I watched everyone go about their business, washing their hands, making dinner, pouring more salt onto their plates. Waiting showed me the ugly face of time, the Dr. Jekyll of the clock. Seconds became minutes, which became hours, which then became days.

Everyone told me that I should be thrilled that there was a heartbeat. However, I wanted to hear the heartbeat constantly, to know that it had not not decided to stop beating mid-way through one of my sentences. The two weeks until my next appointment seemed like the length of a prison term.

I walked around with my hands around my belly, hoping to shield everything, including the air and the sun, from my unborn child and me. My husband had fallen into the *possibly dangerous* category. His callused hands were now weapons with their careless moves, and I could smell the toxins oozing from the oil under his nails. The dust from the car shop coated his skin like a radioactive agent.

Everything started to have lethal edges: the walls, the roads, the television. I licked my finger before I turned the pages of *Moby Dick*, trying to avoid an inevitable slice from the tips of the harpoons, sharpened and ready to maim me at the first signal. I was afraid of any contact, any sudden wrong movement that might cause my body to expel the tiny beat that was barely clinging on as it was.

"I feel like I'll break you if I touch you," my husband said. I was silent and slept on the couch. I thought that he might.

~

I almost made it, with less than two days to go before my scheduled two-week appointment, when the heavy bleeding returned, and I ran out of the bathroom, just in time to receive the call from my mother. My sister had phoned my mother from the admitting desk of the 28 day program, *Right Turn*, in Owings Mills. She had been arrested again, and said she was ready to get help. This time, her body was an aching tube of withdrawal.

My stained underwear dampened the mood as I made another scramble to the doctor's office to hear that the bleeding had stopped again (of course, upon my entrance into his office). I found myself staring at the picture of the doctor's daughters on the bookshelf behind his desk while he finished up his tenth set of notes about me since I had started the pregnancy saga.

All of his daughters had beautiful shiny black hair. The youngest, at least twelve years old, had straight black bangs that cut across her forehead like a short valance. The middle daughter looked to be around fourteen, with a fresh coat of lip-gloss shining across her pouting lips. The oldest, a tall sliver of a girl, stared back at the camera in an independent stare, her eyes like two sharp moons. I was jealous of the triangular stability permeating from the picture, the evenness of the sisters' presence, their lives running like second hands around the strong hourly tick of their father's watch.

"Some women just have a lot of spotting," my doctor stressed. "It should stop around the twelfth week." He continued to explain that I should schedule another appointment for two weeks from then, and I heard myself say *okay*, but what I was really thinking about was him in bed with his wife, a plaid flannel sheet pulled up to his hairy chest. I was trying to determine if he looked into his wife's eyes during their oldest daughter's conception as a lover or as a doctor. I wondered if, during his own children's births, he could pull himself away enough from the delivery table to see the birth process with a new perspective—like it was the first time. Or, did he have to pretend? Did he feel cheated; to already know the outcome before it was his turn?

~

A turkey sub on whole wheat with just mustard from Subway was the first thing that came up, non-discretely in the trashcan under my desk at work. My weight began to go down, and my meals continued to want to come up. The nausea lingered from the moment I woke up until I finally collapsed into the thick pull of sleep. My body was a constant reminder of sickness.

Lunches at the mall with my coworkers became unbearable. I walked around the entire Food Court, reading each menu, hoping some item would not cause the pit of uneasiness in my stomach to erupt. My old favorites, Chicken Teriyaki and Cobb Salad, conjured up images of old septic systems in my mind. Meat made me especially sick, as it seemed to be creeping along the cheap Styrofoam plates in trails of cold grease.

Red meat was particularly evil—I tried not to think about the little pockets of fat hidden in the tissue, or the limp and crusty blood vessels. Chicken was not much better—the texture of the tear between my teeth was the worst part—I could visualize every layer of muscle, each string resistant with its rubbery coating.

I was down to French fries and frozen yogurt. I took tentative bites, like after my wisdom teeth were extracted—slow, careful nibbles. I could feel every tooth rubbing together as I risked swallowing, attempting an uncertain road of digestion. Eating became a chore as difficult as exercising.

~

This time an ex-boyfriend was rubbing my breasts in the dream. I was running my hand over the small of his back as he pinched my nipple with his thumb and forefinger. I woke from the sting, his tongue still wet on my cheek. My breasts were sore and tight like two fresh bruises. I wiped the drool from my cheek and turned my head towards my husband. He was snoring, completely oblivious to my recent mental escapades.

One of my pregnancy books said that dreams of past lovers during pregnancy represent the transition into parenthood. The lovers symbolize the past and appear in dreams to signal the change. I decided I was a special exception to this rule, as my dream lovers were encouraging me to stay in the past. They urged me to find safety in their arms, to remember their familiar smells of young sweat, trendy cologne, and muscles that forever remained firm and tight. I longed for the unharnessed energy rising from their skin like hot steam.

My own body was still young in the dreams, my belly flat and two dimensional. It was the old me in the dreams, pre-pregnant, my hair absent of one single gray, and nothing growing inside of me but ambition. It was my original body, which focused outward then. Then, touch only affected me on a tangible level, and I could enjoy an orgasmic shiver without consequence.

I closed my eyes and tried to go back to sleep, to return to the cracked vinyl backseat of my 1981 Chevy Citation and the arm that was slowing working its way up my thigh.

~

They looked safe from the outside: peaceful scenes of the Madonna and child on the cover, the soft light of evening hovering in the background as the child sleeps on his mother's breast. Opening one book, I expected to hear the melodic tune of a young bluebird. Instead, I found chapters entitled: *When to call the doctor*, *When there IS something wrong*, and *Warning signs*.

Each night I scampered to the pregnancy books, looking up my symptoms in the back pages. The indexes added more stress when I read things like: *Bleeding: Signs of page 29, Bleeding during 1st trimester page 42, Bleeding during 2nd trimester page 68, Bleeding during 3rd trimester page 71, Bleeding with miscarriage page 36, Bleeding during intercourse page 109.*

The books repeated the same words that my doctor did, that some women just experienced more bleeding than others. There wasn't any additional explanation for it, other than it just happened. Each of my symptoms was a part of a long chain of terrible possibilities, like one of those *Make Your Own Adventure* books: to keep bleeding through the 1st

trimester, see page 42, to continue bleeding through the 2nd trimester see page 68, to wake up in tears see page 103, to miscarry again see page 262, to mourn miscarriage read another book.

The books also gave vague statements about cramping: *Many women experience some cramping. If your cramping is strong, call your doctor.* Was my cramping *strong*? I looked up *strong* in the definition indexes, but couldn't find it. I checked again to make sure that I had not missed it between striae distensae (stretch marks) and sudden infant death syndrome (SIDS).

The books hurt me more than they helped me. They increased my anxiety and made me doubt every decision I made. I learned I should have been eating better and doing more consistent exercise. I learned that every ingredient that went into my body was a direct reflection of my responsibility as a mother, and the nail polish fumes and Jolly Ranchers were my badges of neglect. I learned that I should have been more aware of my surroundings, creating a sterile bubble around me at all times. I learned that I needed to be a walking calibrator; I needed to watch every breath that I took.

~

I decided to become a designer of other women's reproductive systems. Instead of comparing the latest hemlines and hairstyles, I kept quotas in a small notebook inside my purse. I noted which pregnant women I saw were smiling and which were having trouble bending over. I made a small circle next to the women who were due within the next two months, their bellies marching ahead of the rest of their bodies. I also documented who had swollen ankles and looked on the edge of exhaustion. It was my new collection, my winter line of choices. The information calmed me, as making a list of the other pregnant women gave me a sense of security that I did not have with my own story. I could sit in the audience and observe, instead of participating in the journey.

    I could dress the other women in my head, folding pregnant stomachs on and off like paper dolls. Some received soft bellies that hid behind cashmere, round breasts and upper arms as warm as bread. Others had tight cotton v-necks, with large belly buttons pushing through like worn quarters. Watching the other pregnant women strut and climb into their cars made them distant objects. It was much easier to dress other people, as the seams were always straighter and the bust-lines always hung just right.

    I was not used to being the one in the midst of the action; the spotlight paused on my body for the rest of the nine months. I was not strong enough to learn the moves, to make it to the end of the crazy pregnancy catwalk. My uterus was a fragile purse, laced together in thin crochet strands. It didn't feel like it could ever hold a growing child, a tiny fetus fighting to remain inside as strand after strand unraveled and dropped out of me into a messy pile of pink yarn.

February

My doctor pulled the Doppler device out of the lowest pocket of his white coat at my ten-week check up. While he squirted some gel onto the bottom of the amplifier, I braced myself for the worst. He pressed it into the lower right side of my abdomen, and I heard what sounded like static. I searched his eyes, trying to read his blank expression.

He moved the Doppler a little to the right, and then pressed it down. The rough static continued, like my childhood television used to when I left it on all night. I listened, looking at the nurse cleaning up the supplies on the counter to see if she paused or missed a beat in her movements. The doctor continued to drag the Doppler back and forth, pressing it down, and then turned it diagonally.

"Not yet," he said, wiping off the gel and slipping the device back into the deep pocket of his coat.

My own heartbeat sped up, the upcoming bad news already pulling its prickly jacket across my body.

"We should be able to hear it next time," he stated.

Next time. That seemed to be the theme of the past few months. I dressed slowly, discouraged, and set up my next appointment for two weeks later at the front desk. I watched the nurse take my file out of a white folder and switch it into a blue one. She noticed my stare.

"Ten weeks," she said, "You've graduated to the blue folder."

The blue folder. I was now out of the early *potential pregnancy* white folder and into the sturdy *definitely pregnant* blue folder. *The blue folder.* Its soft blue color was a huge comfortable couch around me. *The blue folder.* The milestone was more important than getting my driver's license or my marriage certificate.

How many women without children even knew the blue folders existed, high up in their secure place on the top shelf of the filing system, looking out over all of the plain, boring white folders with color-coded tabs? I had never left the white folder during my last pregnancy. How many white folders went uncompleted, eventually ending up being recycled to the next set of unlucky candidates? Perhaps my white folder had contained the records of dozens of other women who had also miscarried before me: *Lynne Davis 8 weeks, Tira Sheldon 6 weeks, Danielle Shuster 7.5 weeks.*

The thought of all those lost pregnancies, those lost hopes, made the white folders seem tainted, wrinkled cases with replaceable tabs, the names constantly changing week after week. I drudged through the next two weeks until my twelve-week appointment. I dreamt about blue pillows and blue windows and a blue whale singing its song in the blue distance.

~

The doctor took out the Doppler again, poured gel on it, and pressed it down into the right side of my abdomen. My hands pulled into clenched fists, and I turned my head to the side, the same way I turned my head when I got a blood test. Somehow, not looking helped to alleviate the worry, not seeing what was happening made it someone else's procedure.

He held the Doppler still, and I heard the same static sound from my last appointment. He moved the Doppler to the left and the sound continued; a constant hum of machine and echo. I tilted my head around enough to see my doctor's tan hand twisting the Doppler towards the middle of my pelvis. I started to re-dress myself in my head, ready for the news that there was still not a heartbeat, and I would be demoted back to the white folder.

After a couple of minutes of maneuvering the Doppler around, the doctor lowered it down below my pelvic hairline, and I heard a difference in the sound. There was a faint rumble, like thunder or a distant train.

The nurse patted my arm.

"It's low," the doctor said and smiled.

However, I barely heard him because I was looking past him, past the nurse with her warm hand on my arm, past the poster on the wall of Lupus and its symptoms, past the Sheetrock of the next examining room, past the receptionist's window, and past the lobby with its glass display case of doctors' names and office suites. I was already out of the parking lot, the tree lined entrance, and the front gate of the hospital, trying to follow the sound of the rumbling to its origin. All I knew was that it was somewhere far outside of this office and me. It was coming from a place I had never been.

~

I was afraid that if I blinked too much the heartbeat might stop. I needed reassurance that it had not already stopped, just twenty minutes after the exam, as I veered off Joppa Road and pulled into Babies R Us. I asked the customer service clerk to direct me towards the correct aisle to find the prenatal heartbeat listeners. She didn't know what I was talking about, so I was left pacing the aisles until I found them crammed next to two shelves of discounted unscented wipes. The heartbeat listeners resembled old Sony Walkmans, with attached headphones and small amplifiers that extended from the back of each case.

I bought extra batteries and tore open the package as soon as I was back in the car. After I skimmed the directions, I assembled the heartbeat listener and placed it directly on my stomach. The directions suggested using the device in a quiet area to keep any interference to a minimum. I figured the parking lot of Towson Place Shopping Center wasn't too noisy, so I gave it a shot.

With my pants around my knees and the headphones on, I moved the heartbeat listener over the spot where the doctor had found the heartbeat—in the middle of my lower pelvis. At first, I heard loud static, and then some faint gurgling. Reading the instructions again, I learned that the gurgling was only my own stomach digesting. The instructions stated that a heartbeat would be *faint and quick, like distant clapping*. I couldn't hear anything but static and my stomach growling. I was starting to sweat from the heat that was rising in the closed car, so I rolled the window down a bit, and suddenly the heartbeat listener picked up the steady rhythm of a person walking towards my car. I turned to the left to see one of the Sisters from the Catholic high school where I used to teach headed my way.

I sunk down as low as I could in my seat. I felt like I had just been caught making out with a boy. I yanked my pants up and slid the headphones down around my neck. Maybe she would think I was just listening to Amy Grant. I sunk down even lower and readied myself for my due reprimand. Instead, I heard her thick soles continue past the car. I wiped the sweat from my brow and decided to resume my heartbeat search at home.

In the quiet of the bedroom I tuned into the dog barking, a passing plane, and the ring of the telephone, but no heartbeat. The loud sounds of my digestive system had most likely scared the fetus to death. I could only imagine the world that my baby was living in, full of half chewed French fries, yappy dogs, and alarm clocks.

Each night I tried to hear the heartbeat, but without luck. I moved the heartbeat listener over my entire belly, searching for the beat that would calm my anxiety. Once, I thought I heard it for a second, but then the beating became louder and louder, and I realized that it was only a motorcycle revving by the house.

~

I couldn't decide which entrée to order, hidden behind the long tri-fold menu of Carrabba's Italian Grill in Overlea. Each linguine noodle was calling my name with the promise of seasoned comfort. The picture of the Chicken Alfredo made my mouth water, and I couldn't take my eyes off the description of the Eggplant Parmesan with fresh tomato basil sauce. I wanted to celebrate the day, the first day that I had not been overwhelmed by nausea, the first day that my stomach would accept instead of repel.

Finally, I decided on the Portobello Mushroom Ravioli in a light cream sauce. Ten minutes later, my fork split a pasta pocket down the middle, and I watched thin pieces of mushroom roll out into the buttery sauce. The sauce ran over the grape leaves painted daintily around the edge of the plate.

It was heaven. The hesitation in my belly was only a slight whisper as I sunk my teeth into the tender dough. I wanted to devour every scrap of flavor, even the parsley sprinkles scattered around the pasta, as well as the adorable waiter who kept bringing me more bread without a flinch. I could have licked his six o'clock stubble or bitten his lips until they bled. Instead, I asked him to bring the dessert tray and to tell me the names of each choice three times. I pictured my finger dotting his chest with chocolate as he repeated, "Tiramisu," "Mocha Cannoli," "Neapolitan Torte," and "Raspberry Cheesecake."

~

I said goodbye to the days of crackers and lemonade and hello to the hours of pasta, chocolate, and ice cream. The pounds seemed to increase by the hour. At first, I could barely button my pants, and then I couldn't close them at all.

Strangers stared at my stomach like it was a third boob. They weren't sure if I was pregnant or just had a beer belly. I stared at it too, in between gulps of Golden Grahams. I touched it and tried to move my hand across it gracefully, the way I saw the pregnant women at the mall do. However, all I felt was a bloated gut and the tight strap of my underwear digging into my skin. I was stuck wearing my old sweat pants and leggings to work. I needed to get some maternity clothes soon, or I was going to resemble a Richard Simmons' *Sweatin' to the Oldies* video participant.

 I thought I would gain confidence with the growth of my stomach. I thought more space would equal more peace. I had believed that if I could touch my growing belly, I could finally believe that the baby was growing too. Instead, I felt like the same person, just larger. In fact, I think the fat cells opened up even more room for my anxiety. My worries now had a larger square footage for their breeding. They flipped and somersaulted throughout my body. I just hoped that they were staying outside of my uterus, that they left this baby alone and continued their straddling and squatting down my legs and into the pads of my feet.

~

* I pulled the silky slips out of my mother's top drawer and ran my fingers along the snug elastic. The slips were "adult" colors—light beige, cream, ochre, and sheer. All of them were hues not found in my own closet, where red, yellow and pink swayed like short kites from the homemade wood bar wedged up too high for me to reach.*

* I draped the slips over my ten-year-old body and looked at my short legs through the sheer material. My skin was different through the gauze, sexy and tan. I moved my hands over my legs, feeling the silky panels glide back and forth like water.*

I day-dreamed what it would be like to fit into the slips one day, with a tall body, curvy white hips, and long shaven legs. Of course, I always placed a handsome man in the background, holding a drink, a coconut shell filled with yellow umbrellas and sparkly green toothpicks.

I slipped the bras on next, tightening the back hooks until the straps didn't fall off my shoulders. I filled the empty front cups with pantyhose and posed in front of the mirror. I wanted to look like the teenage girls in the older Sunday school class with their mysterious cleavage peeking out of the tops of their sweaters. I knew life would be exciting with breasts. Everything would be more alluring. Everything would feel like silk against my body. I couldn't imagine ever having a bad day if I had two beautiful breasts to keep me company.

I had to get a stool to reach my mother's dresses. They hung up so high that I usually waited until she was outside talking to the next-door neighbor to climb up and touch them. I ran my hands back and forth against the dresses. They were the colors of night; of places I had never seen, of make-up, hair spray, and high heeled shoes. I especially loved the ones with belts, silver or gold buckles that tightened around my middle and accentuated my pantyhose stuffed bras. I slipped my feet into her high heeled shoes, shuffled back and forth across the carpeted bedroom, and watched my reflection prance by in the mirror. I longed for the day I would fit into a 36B, or the night I would slip on three-inch pumps. I would be the belle of the ball, not the shy girl who stuttered when her teacher called on her, or the girl who tried to find an empty seat on the bus.

~

At first, I just walked around the store, checking out the different styles and sizes. Then I started touching the clothes, running my finger along the huge pleated waists, trying to picture myself actually wearing these awkward triangles of fabric.

The sales clerk helped me pick out a pair of jeans and a couple of cotton shirts. There was a pouch of stretchy cotton material stitched into the stomach of the jeans. I tried the jeans on first, pulling the stretchy belly over my small gut and tightening the drawstring to keep the pants up. It looked like I had a kangaroo pouch.

I pulled a red shirt over the jeans and stared back at the dressing room mirror. I didn't even look pregnant. The shirt covered up the stretchy pouch so that it just looked like I was wearing jeans and a baggy top. I stepped out into the bright light of the store and smiled at the sales clerk.

"They fit," I told her. In fact, they felt really comfortable.

"Now try it on with this." The sales clerk handed me a soft pillow the size of a dinner plate. I stepped back into the dressing room and pushed the pillow into the belly pocket of the maternity jeans.

The shirt immediately puffed out and there stood an obviously pregnant woman. This couldn't be me. I would never get this big. I looked at myself from all angles in the mirror and saw a pregnant woman staring back at me for the first time. I opened the dressing room shutters to get a better view in the full-length mirror.

The sales clerk looked up from the ticket she was currently marking down with a black marker.

"You'll get much bigger," she said. "You'll probably want to go with the next size up."

~

The doctor measured my belly. He was a quick tailor, pulling out the measuring tape and lining it up from my pelvis to my lower chest. As he read off the measurements to the nurse and she jotted them down in my folder, I imagined a transparent dress with flesh colored smocking down the front and sleeves that overlapped like wet petals. It would be my own version of a temple garment, the soft white underwear that my mother slipped into each morning, the constant reminders of her devotion to God, a hidden wall between herself and the rest of the world.

I originally heard about the garments in Sunday school lessons, subtle references to the sacred clothes that all faithful Mormon adults acquired after they promised to be faithful to God for eternity. It was a whispered topic even when I was an active member, as the garments represented a secret world that no one could enter until adulthood, provided in a ritual ceremony at the temple. My mother had received hers when I was in high school, finally getting the bishop's recommendation to seal herself to the church, without my father, at the temple in Washington, D.C.

I was curious and confused. I didn't know if the garments provided protection, like my long underwear, a layer of warmth around the body, or if they were actually spiritual lingerie, snug cotton that rubbed against breasts and pubic hair, God's hidden peep show underneath turtlenecks and long skirts.

I decided to secretly wear my own garment of pregnancy. It would be my own reminder of my devotion to this child. Every time the doctor lengthened the measuring tape to the next black notch, I would see the dress expanding, my belly stretching forward with the clicks of the tape.

~

I still doubted my sister's desire to stay clean, even when she completed the inpatient 28 day program and called my parents to see if they could help to move her into a halfway house on Linwood Avenue. I went along for the ride, to support her move from one physical space to another, her body the playing piece making its way around the board after being dealt a GET OUT OF JAIL FREE card. Her stuff consisted of:

- *a 13" TV*
- *a set of mismatched flower print twin sheets*
- *a pillow with a faded pink pillowcase*
- *an old clock radio*
- *two pictures (one of the family in front of the Christmas tree two years before and one of her fat orange cat on my parents' couch)*
- *a garbage bag full of clothes*
- *3 pairs of old beat up shoes*
- *a reading lamp*
- *a shoe box of bath items (which contained shampoo and conditioner, a wide toothed comb, deodorant, toothbrush and toothpaste, and Clean and Clear acne wash)*
- *her Narcotics Anonymous little white book (the condensed version of*

the NA Basic Text)

I skimmed through the little white book during our slow drive down I-83, the beams and oil of the city gradually growing around the tight safety holds of the interstate's jersey walls, as my sister kept her gaze out the window. My sister had penned her sponsor's name and phone number in the front of the book in black letters and numbers. It still looked like the handwriting of a child to me with the perfectly round o's helping to hold the hard stems of the d's and p's. I found the recovery steps near the beginning of the book, after the preface, *How It Works*:

1. *We admitted that we were powerless over our addiction, that our lives had become unmanageable.*
2. *We came to believe that a Power greater than ourselves could restore us to sanity.*
3. *We made a decision to turn our will and our lives over to the care of God as we understood Him.*
4. *We made a searching and fearless moral inventory of ourselves.*
5. *We admitted to God, to ourselves, and to another human being the exact nature of our wrongs.*
6. *We were entirely ready to have God remove all these defects of character.*
7. *We humbly asked Him to remove our shortcomings.*
8. *We made a list of all persons we had harmed, and became willing to make amends to them all.*
9. *We made direct amends to such people wherever possible, except when*

10. *We continued to take personal inventory and when we were wrong promptly admitted it.*
11. *We sought through prayer and meditation to improve our conscious contact with God as we understood Him, praying only for knowledge of His will for us and the power to carry that out.*
12. *Having had a spiritual awakening as a result of these steps, we tried to carry this message to addicts, and to practice these principles in all our affairs.*

My father carried in the TV and her bag of clothes. My mother took her lamp and the bath items. My sister went in empty handed. I rushed past everyone and headed straight for the bathroom, my bladder about to burst from the pressure. The bathroom ceiling was peeling, and the flakes were sprinkled in patches across the cracked brown floor tile, among hundreds of cigarette burns and different colored pieces of hair. I threw two pieces of toilet paper down on the toilet seat and barely made it before my bladder relaxed. While I sat on the toilet, I read a typed note taped crookedly inside a cheap wood frame, positioned with a bent nail on the opposite wall:

Rules for Recovery- *This means you!*

1. *NO drugs*
2. *NO drinking*
3. *Leave relationships alone for one year*
4. *Pray*

(continued from previous page: *to do so would injure them or others.*)

5. Get a sponsor
6. Practice spiritual principles, esp. honesty and willingness
7. Help out the newcomer
8. Take the cotton out of your ears and put it in your mouth—**LISTEN**
9. Get a network
10. Follow your program!

The sign was not for me to read. It was too obvious that I was only a visitor here. The scratched up walls seemed to be saying, "You'll be leaving soon," as I met everyone back in my sister's room, the first room on the left of the second floor.

There wasn't anything left to do after all of my sister's belongings found a spot in the middle of her new room. We returned to the living room, standing out like square pegs. There were two other residents sitting on the couch watching *Jerry Springer*. They were both thin black women in their late thirties. They smiled at us, the way you smile at a relative you do not really like, just because you have to.

"Well, I guess that's it," my mother said, trying to sound like she was dropping my sister off for a week at Girl Scout camp.

"Yup," my sister stated, without any emotion.

"Do you want to go get something to eat?" My mother turned to my father and me.

"Sure," I said for the both of us, though I knew no one was hungry. We decided on Nacho Mammas, where we would just sit and stare at our larger than life burritos.

We awkwardly headed out the narrow doorway, and as I turned around to say goodbye to my sister, I saw one of the women on the couch get up and walk into the kitchen. A small pregnant belly popped out from beneath her button-down shirt. I hadn't noticed she was pregnant before because of the way she was sitting. It was hard to tell how far along she was, because she was so thin.

The next day my sister casually mentioned that both of the other women living in the halfway house had H.I.V.

"They're shooters," she said, like they were twins or late risers.

I pictured the pregnant woman's tiny arms, the loose denim shirt buttoned tight around her wrists. Then I thought of her in that old stale bathroom, naked in the shower with the paint falling from the ceiling, as the steam from the hot water covered up her needle marks and the moldy blue shower curtain hid the tiny belly that somehow kept on growing.

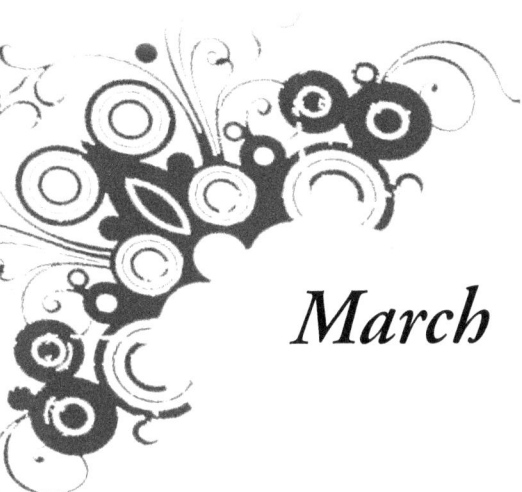

March

It was an early dating game, just like *M.A.S.H. (Mansion, Apartment, Shack, and House)* or *Friendship, Courtship, Marriage, Love, Hate.* The idea of a baby was just as abstract. The names were part of the formula: one boy name, one girl name, just like us.

I started writing different names down as my eighteen week appointment approached. It was the point where I could get another ultrasound. I wrote the names in cursive, in bubble letters, in blocks, on a slant, on lined paper, and on napkins. I looked at the names, trying to picture a face to match each. The words were still abstract, the letters just decorations on the page.

I practiced the name writing exercise that I assigned to my students when I was teaching at the Catholic school, which was to use all of the five senses to describe a name.

My boy's name should sound like strong talons, like the pull of a deep root from the ground. It should smell like sand, and the cement mix of a basement. It should taste like steak, a thick Western fry, and Grandma's mashed potatoes with extra butter. It should feel like a horse's mane, a rope across the palm. It needed to look bold and unafraid, with dark eyes that would tell the future.

My girl's name should sound like chimes, like the creak of a porch door. It should smell like lily of the valley, of lemon Pledge and misty rain. It should taste like phyllo pastry layers, crisp lettuce among homemade croutons. It should be an acquired taste, like sun-dried tomatoes and capers. It should feel like linen, the long tassels of an Oriental rug across a wood floor. It needed to look like a piece of mica shining through the grass, like an antique earring lost among the rafters.

~

I watched the other patients as they entered the radiology office on their tiptoes and then signed in on the three-page waiting list. The receptionist argued with a woman on crutches about her lack of a referral. I looked to my left at the man sitting next to me, his face caved in with wrinkles, as he gagged and continued to drink a tall glass of chalky liquid.

I pretended to read a six-month-old issue of *Gardener's Delight* and then a two-year-old issue of *Exotic Travel Locations*. What I was really doing was trying to guess whose number was up, who was there to be officially diagnosed with lung cancer, who was there to get a routine mammogram, and who was there to double check because things *just didn't seem right*. We all sat silently, like an unlikely group of civilians waiting for the draft pick.

Finally, a technician called my name and led me into the back room. She looked like she was barely fourteen years old, as she snapped her cinnamon gum and looked down at my folder. She opened the curtain to a tiny dressing room with six miniature lockers and a small bench and instructed me to take off my clothes and put on the blue cotton gown that was waiting on the bench, wrapped up in plastic like a new shirt. After I changed, I stepped out into the women's waiting area, where there were three cushioned chairs and three end tables positioned in a horseshoe formation. Large Kleenex boxes and magazines fanned themselves across the tables.

There was a poster on the wall next to me with drawings of a fetus at each week of a pregnancy. At eighteen weeks, my current week, it looked like a shriveled version of a baby, with a huge broccoli head and a body like an arthritic hand. I couldn't believe that there was something inside of me that looked like the baby in the diagram. I scanned back over the former weeks, at the tadpole with the bulging eyes encased in a sac of blood, and then ahead to six months and saw an actual little baby starting to fill out the uterus with its growing extremities. I traced my finger over the mini-baby for my week. It looked so alone, cut down to a close-up shot in its tight picture box, with only one dark eye visible from this side profile and its fists curled up into small knots. It probably didn't even know that it was alive, its heartbeat going on autopilot, its limbs drifting back and forth like seaweed in the warm fluid.

The technician appeared again and said my name, and I followed her into an examination room where she typed my information onto a keyboard while I climbed up on the table. Without speaking, she pulled my gown open, poured gel onto my stomach from a container that looked like it used to contain ketchup and began to move the transducer across it. I looked at the screen in anticipation.

I saw a few blinks of movement and what looked like a chubby belly.

"Is that the stomach?" I asked, thrilled at my own diagnosis.

"No," the technician responded flatly. "That's the head."

I sat still, as she told me to, and waited to recognize the next body part as she kept making tiny measurements of the baby's head from her keyboard station. She kept clicking and enlarging the circles across its head, causing light blue lines to climb up and down the dark screen.

"What are you doing now?" I asked her.

"Just measuring," she replied, annoyed, like I was interrupting her train of thought.

Inside the dark circle of the head were a few oddly shaped forms. She measured each of them and then typed into the keyboard. I started to worry. Did the baby have tumors growing in its brain? She kept measuring and clicking. This couldn't be normal.

"Is this normal?" I hesitantly asked.

"You'll have to ask your doctor," she snapped back. "We don't read the ultrasounds. We just take them."

"Do you have kids?" I asked.

"Nope," she replied with a heavy chomp of her cinnamon gum.

I thought that I saw an arm waving in frantic circles, but then it was gone and the screen blurred.

Half an hour later, she was still measuring. She told me to turn on my side and brought in an older technician who must have been all of twenty-one years old. I knew there had to be something wrong. My child was probably deformed. There were tumors everywhere. I was pregnant with conjoined twins. Neither of the technicians would look me in the eye. They just kept clicking and pushing the transducer into my abdomen, so hard that I thought I was going to wet myself.

After an hour, the older technician finally put the transducer down and told me I would probably have to come back for another ultrasound.

"Why?" I gulped.

"We can't see everything," she said.

"What do you mean?" I asked, the tears filling up the cups of my bottom eye lids.

"Only your doctor can read the results," she finalized. Now I knew there had to be a problem.

"Can you at least tell me if it's a boy or a girl?" I pleaded.

"I'll try," she huffed and shoved the transducer even further into my abdomen.

"Your baby is really not cooperating today," she added.

I was already picturing the baby's medical file growing to the size of the yellow pages, with the labels: *Uncooperative, Deformed, A Never Before Seen Case*. I watched the screen, looking for some sign of a penis, or some sign of no penis, but all I could see were lava lamp shapes that kept blending into one another. The older technician twisted the transducer to the left. I felt a few drops of urine escape from between my legs.

"I think I might have seen something," she stated, "but it won't uncross its legs." I looked at the screen, trying to tell if the two gray shadows I was looking at were legs.

"I think it might be a boy, but I'm not certain," she finally declared and punched PRINT on the computer before tearing off the picture like it was a gasoline receipt. She handed the picture to me and told me that I could finally go to the bathroom and get dressed. It felt like a warm river, the urine gushing out of me for at least five minutes. The whole time I just stared at the picture, the thin edges already starting to wrinkle in my hands. It was a side shot, a profile. There was a definite head, a nose, a mouth, the slope of a neck, and the slight curve of a chest. Above the chest, small crescents of fingers poked out above a tiny palm. *My baby.* I tried to say it aloud, but I could only mouth it.

~

The cake was waiting in the middle of the kitchen table when I arrived at my mother's house after the ultrasound. *Congratulations! It's a _____!* beamed in bright yellow letters across the cake's white whipped frosting. My grandparents popped their heads around the corner of the dining room. The next-door neighbor stepped away from the sink and smiled. I shuffled in as everyone crowded around me to hear the news.

"They're not sure," I looked down at my feet. "It might be a boy, but they're not sure. And I have to go back for another ultrasound, and they won't tell me why."

Everyone took a step back, caught off guard, and there were a couple of seconds of uncomfortable silence before pretend smiles resurfaced.

"Oh, I'm sure everything is fine," my mother stated and ran back into the kitchen to finish cutting the carrots.

"They didn't tell you *anything*?" my grandmother asked.

"No, just that they couldn't see everything," I told her, trying to keep the tears from running out of my eyes.

"Those doctors. Half the time they don't know what they're doing," my grandfather chimed in. "They made me go back three times for my last chest scan."

"I hope that's it," I said, as he put his arm around my shoulder and pinched my ear.

"Let's eat," my mother called out from the kitchen, and we all proceeded to the safe distraction of food. I only ate a few bites, as I was looking around at everyone else's paper plates, at the plastic forks shoveling up food and returning to the plates within seconds for more. After dinner, my mother cut the cake for me. I took a thin sliver. The cake tasted sour, like my stomach. The party ended early as the skies darkened, and my grandparents decided to hurry home to beat the upcoming storm.

~

That weekend I debated about what to do with my anxiety. I was a walking nerve, a sharp question mark. My whole body was a complete pit of fear. It felt like I was living and not living at the same time. I continued to go through the motions of life: food, sleep, air, but none of it felt substantial. What was I supposed to feel when I didn't know if this baby would make it into the next month?

I decided to stay on the couch, watching cable, finding every show I could about disasters: hurricanes, fires, earthquakes, and floods. For some reason I enjoyed the enormity of the destruction, my own trauma taking a backseat to the thousands of lives affected by each disaster. I recorded the flood episode on *The Learning Channel* where an old woman wades through her house, moving a floating board from her china cabinet out of the way, so that she can walk through the stagnant pool that used to be her living room. I wondered if the cabinet had immediately fallen over into the rising water, or if it had tried to stay mounted, to hold its breath until the wood would not absorb another drop. How long did the nails hold before the water ripped them from their grooves, the white china immediately crushed like eggshells?

I tried to imagine my own house in a flood. Would the dogs be able to escape through the doggy door, to swim to higher ground with their bruised paws? Would I be able to save my writing disks and binders scattered randomly throughout the rooms? What would I take if I only had time to grab one thing? Would I take my laptop, a photo album, or my plastic bin full of old yearbooks and school awards? What would I do if I didn't have time to take anything from the house? Would I be able to live with just myself as the survivor, all proof of my history destroyed within seconds?

~

The following Monday I called my doctor and described the ultrasound ordeal to the nurse.

"Ah. Uh. We'll give you a call when we receive the pictures," she casually said.

"When will that be?" I begged.

"Within the week."

The doctor's office was in the same building as the radiology lab. How could it possibly take a week to deliver the pictures 50 feet down the hall?

"It's standard delivery time," the nurse recited, as if it was the obvious answer to my question.

I hung up. What standard were they going by, the standard for causing a nervous breakdown among their patients?

Luckily, the doctor called me back the next day, as I was close to scheduling an electric shock therapy session.

"They just couldn't see the four chambered heart," he said, surprised at my concern. "It happens a lot—sometimes the baby's position won't let them see a certain view. We will schedule you for another ultrasound at twenty-two weeks. The baby should be a lot bigger by then."

"But everything looks okay?" I pleaded.

"Yes, it looks fine," he confirmed.

It was too quick of an answer. He couldn't have looked at all of my ultrasound views. Did he miss the cluster of tumors, the five legs, and the stomach shaped like a rotten green pepper?

"I'll see you again after the next ultrasound," he said. "Goodbye."

I was supposed to feel relieved. The thought that everything might possibly be alright crept into my mind, but then I quickly dismissed it.

~

The four chambered heart sounded like an Edgar Allen Poe story, each chamber containing the remains of a lunatic's rampage:

The first chamber was a parlor. I could see a dark green chaise lounge and bourbon glasses waiting on the top of a chrome bar. There was dust along the arteries of this room, a faint film of white that might leave enough proof for the lifting of one guilty fingerprint.

The second room was a music chamber with a black grand piano, its foot pedals covered with thick cobwebs. The silence in this room was deafening, the harsh contrast after a piercing sound has been recently released. Only the ceiling of this chamber held any clue, its throat swollen from swallowing so much grief.

The library chamber's shelves climbed every wall, filled with old copies of Old Man and the Sea and Moby Dick. It would take three long years to review every page in this room, to place a magnifying lens to every vessel and nerve. The books waited in their alphabetical places, closed tight like mute witnesses.

The final room, the bedroom chamber, had a maple canopy, with high mattresses and yellow mosquito netting draping down from the frame. This was the most suspicious room, with slash marks through the pink silk sheets of the bed. This room smelled the most like death.

Only, in my story, no one could enter to search for the corpse, as the chambers were inaccessible, deep inside, closed off from detectives and investigators. In my story, the corpse remained unnamed, without recognition. It was neither man nor woman, just an object out of reach, permanently hidden from view.

~

I got out of the week long fundraising conference in Houston by declaring that my doctor had forbidden any travel. He actually never said it, but it sounded good as an excuse. I pictured the nightmare in my head: me, on a stretcher, blood soaking between my thighs during a training session as my coworkers called for an ambulance to rush me to the nearest hospital. There, a cold doctor in a stiff white coat would confirm that it was another miscarriage. I could see the sterile hospital room, my bloody clothes in the corner, and the dim light from the bathroom casting a green glow on the white tiles of the floor.

My home for the week was up front in the lobby, answering the phone and twiddling my thumbs. I didn't mind. Boredom was definitely a step up above fear. However, after two days of Mahjong on the computer, I broke down and brought in *Moby Dick* and my writing journal.

After about an hour into the history of the sperm whale from the dawn of time, I decided to take a break from reading and pulled out the short story contest ad that one of my writing friends had recently mailed to me. Artscape, the city's summer arts festival, was holding a short story contest, and the only requirement for the story was that it had to be less than 1000 words. I set the ad next to the computer.

1000 words. It wasn't enough words to tell my life story. It was too many words for a poem. I thought about the past few months. Should I write about the baby, my sister, my uncle, or the hunt for an unattainable whale? I needed a teacher to help me find a strong topic sentence, to link our lives into logical words. I knew it was not possible; our worlds were all in limbo as we moved into the next unknown stage, one unsure foot in front of the other. It was the in-between, the transition, which held us together. *Halfway*: that was the word. I began the story.

Part Three

Almost

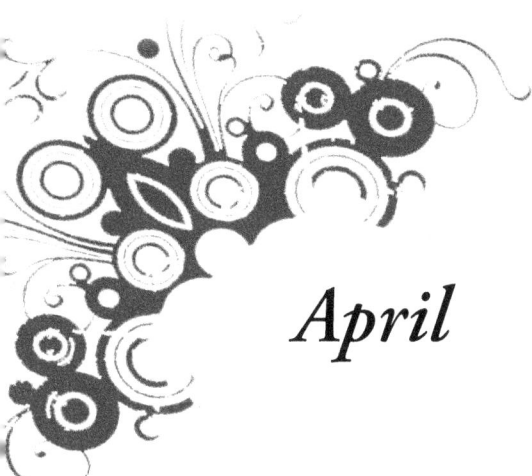

April

I purposely scheduled my next ultrasound for 7:00 a.m. in the morning. That way, I didn't have to spend the entire day sitting around, waiting, and biting my fingernails. I prayed that the rude technician from the last ultrasound would not be on the early shift.

Luckily, the waiting room was still a ghost town at that time of the day, so it was only a matter of minutes before a chubby technician with Hello Kitty scrubs called me into the back and escorted me into the dressing room. As I was changing, I noticed a pile of questionnaire cards and an input box in my dressing room cubicle. It was the standard questionnaire: *How would you rate your visit on a scale of 1-10? Was your technician professional? Was your technician timely? Feel free to make comments.*

Yes! I fished out a pen from my purse and went to town, describing my previous terrible ultrasound experience. My essay took up all of the pre-printed lines and continued onto the back of the card. I placed exclamation marks at the end of every statement, underlining the sentence: <u>The technician made me feel like there was something wrong with my baby!</u>

Boy, did I ever take pleasure in the complaint card, hoping the technician's supervisor would soon be pulling her aside: *What is this I hear about you being insensitive to a patient? How dare you make that patient feel insecure and worried! Get your belongings and take the first bus home!*

I smiled at the thought of her riding the bus home, still in her white lab coat, wishing she had been nicer to me as her career went down the drain. I saw her opening up her front door, throwing her dismissal notice onto the pile of unpaid bills on her kitchen table, and finding her Beta fish belly-up in the round bowl next to her microwave.

The Hello Kitty technician was much nicer and explained what she was doing while I watched the screen.

"Look there," she pointed to the middle of the screen, where I saw a crooked cross expanding, then releasing. "Can you see the four chambers of the heart?"

I stared as she measured and typed into the computer. The cross wiggled and continued to puff in and out. I could definitely see the four chambers, the cross separating the heart in asymmetrical cuts. It was a child's rendition of a heart, the off-center dimensions and curved lines too arbitrary to be accidental.

"Can you tell if it's a girl or a boy?" I asked.

"I'll try," she said, pressing the transducer down on my abdomen and moving it to the right a couple of inches from my belly button. She pushed it down even more, and then twisted it to the left.

"I see a turtle," she smiled.

"Where?" I asked, looking frantically at the screen for a turtle, for a hardened shell or a snapping head.

"There," she pointed, and I suddenly saw a gray speckled shadow of a small turtle, its head peeking out from under the two shy lumps of a shell.

"Looks like a boy to me," she stated and pulled the transducer away a final time. The turtle disappeared from the screen.

"Are you sure?" I asked.

"Well, we can't promise, but I'd say 95%."

I couldn't believe it! She had found a four chambered heart and a turtle! And it was only 8:10 a.m. in the morning! My adrenaline was pumping at full speed, and I still had a full day left at work. It didn't matter what I had to do that day; nothing could break my mood. In fact, I couldn't stop smiling. I grinned the whole way back to the office, and my cheeks were burning by the time I reached the parking lot. The reception door bell rang as I walked in, announcing, "It's a turtle!"

~

I was beyond self conscious as I walked into the first *Moms in Motion* class, a swim session for pregnant women at the Maryland Athletic Center in Timonium. I had my new maternity bathing suit in my duffle bag and was still raw from just shaving my legs and bikini area right before the class.

Once I was in the pool area, I immediately saw two other women who had to be in the class. They were petite women, with tiny soccer balls fastened to the front of their bodies. Neither woman had any puffiness under her eyes or extra cellulite at the tops of her thighs. One was a brunette and the other was a blonde, but both had the same beautiful long hair swept up in sleek ponytails, and similar diamond rings, at least a couple of carats on each princess cut. The brunette had a dark red bathing suit that highlighted the tan she was remarking she had just picked up in Bermuda. The blonde was modestly explaining that she and her husband wouldn't be taking any time for a vacation because they were adding on an eight room addition for the new baby and wanted to be home at all times to supervise the messy contractors.

I passed the pool area and went into the locker room in the back of the building to change. I couldn't avoid seeing myself in the dressing room mirror: my belly was at least three times the size of either of the women's bellies in the pool, my legs were as thick as tree stumps, and the bathing suit that I thought looked so cute in the store suddenly resembled a giant tablecloth. I waddled from the locker room to the pool, stepped down into the water, and slid over into the corner of the shallow end. The water lifted the weight off my stomach and hid my figure. I felt lighter, and relieved.

The instructor led us back and forth across the pool, doing different moves with each lap: pendulum swings, rocking horses, and hamstring curls. It was a bizarre sight, as we were a group of bloated synchronized swimmers. After the aerobics part was over, I followed the other women out of the big pool and into the therapy pool. We pulled Styrofoam noodles out of the bin and floated around on them. It was very relaxing, like lounging in a big bathtub with our bellies all hidden under the water. Then, we formed a circle, the noodles tucked under our arms to support our weight, and discussed due dates, jobs, ultrasounds, and baby names.

It was a forced club—*Moms in Motion*—with no other commonality than our growing stomachs. Watching the women who were further along, the ones who were coming close to their due dates, was like previewing graduation as a junior, viewing the seniors like they knew everything in the world. I envied the eight and nine month women. They were *almost* there. The urgency of their upcoming dates alone made them smarter and prettier.

For the rest of my pregnancy I would see them like that: one step ahead, due in May, June, and July. They were early girls who would beat the heat of the summer, and leave me in the deep end of the pool, waiting for a date in late August. They were the beautiful girls with full bellies and cute ponytails, beautiful girls who were not quite yet mothers.

~

The brochure was set up like a college course catalogue. I debated over the electives. Should we take *Infant CPR* and *Infant Care*? Did we need *Childbirth I* and *II*? We definitely needed to sign up for *Lamaze*! It felt like every class was a pre-requisite for fit parenting. Two hundred and fifty dollars later I had us signed up for *Childbirth I* and *II* (*Lamaze* was included in *Part II*), *Infant CPR*, *Anesthesia*, and *Breastfeeding Basics*. The classes met in the evenings from 7:00 to 9:30 p.m. I couldn't wait for the classes to begin, but my husband seemed much less enthusiastic about them.

When the day of the first class rolled around I anxiously approached the auditorium full of at least fifty other pregnant women and their partners. My swollen ankles were aching so much that I barely made the walk from the parking lot to the lecture hall at the hospital without needing to stop for a break. We grabbed a seat in the back, and I waited for the throbbing in my feet to subside.

The first session of Childbirth I was an up close and personal look at the actual birth process. It featured a film from the seventies which documented the birth experience of two different couples. The first couple opted for natural childbirth without pain management, while the second couple had elected for an epidural during the labor.

"Look at the couple who chooses the natural method," one of the two instructors pointed out before the film started. She had long gray hair and no make-up.

"Look at the way the husband helps to guide his wife through the process with his support and reassurance," the other instructor reinforced. She had short gray hair and no make-up.

The *natural method* pair was a hippie couple in the process of birthing their fifth child when the film opened. The wife pulled her torso into a tight curve as the contractions started. Her husband massaged her back, gently stroking her waist length hair away from her face, and constantly kissed her nose and forehead. He was so close to the camera that even I could smell his pot breath through the film reel. The instructors sighed, obviously admiring his close attention to his wife. I thought about how I would probably slap my husband if he smothered me like that during labor, as I couldn't even stand to feel his rough leg hair in the middle of the night. When I was sick, his hands touching me anywhere was repulsive.

The couple continued to make out for the next fifteen minutes of the film, through various sets of contractions, and then the pushing began. The woman began to breathe heavier, in long sighs, and her eyelids started to pull down with the pressure. Her husband continued to massage her through it all.

"Look at me!" he smiled, and she responded like a trained dog.

"Look at me! Right here! Look at me!" his voice deepened as the ten-pound baby crowned between her tiny thighs.

The film cut to the second couple and quickly focused to a close up of the husband, his two-foot afro almost touching the ceiling of the delivery room. He pleaded directly to the camera: "For God's sake, give her the drugs! It's real ugly, man, real ugly!"

The camera panned back to the wife. Her hair was falling out of her ponytail into a dreaded mess on the top of her head. She gritted her teeth and growled at the lens.

The film skipped through a rough splice and the wife was already pushing, her hands gripping a large metal bar positioned above the delivery bed like a high-wire beam. She was squatting under the bar, hanging on for dear life.

"Get this thing out of me," the wife screeched at the top of her lungs. "Get it out!"

Finally, dark curls began to appear between her legs. The film ended with another close up of the husband's shocked face, his eyebrows raised all the way up to his hairline.

I looked around the auditorium. All the men in the room were examining their watches and re-tying their shoes. The women were all staring at the men.

"The power of the *mind*," the instructor with short gray hair said as she concluded the session with an emphasis on *mind* for dramatic effect. The instructors turned to each other and smiled. For a minute, I thought they might be readying for an encore.

On the way home I couldn't stop thinking about the metal bar above the second woman's delivery bed. It was just like a gymnasium bar, a bar that a small child would hold onto for as long as she could without letting go.

~

The layout of our bathroom was so tight that I had to turn sideways to squeeze by the sink as I approached my sixth month. We decided it was time to do our "big" project, to remodel the bathroom so that I could get to the toilet. My father recommended the help of a handyman he was currently using to do some roof repairs, a guy from my sister's NA home group in Canton.

The handyman came over to discuss the plans and stressed the fact that he always left his work sites by four p.m. to attend his daily NA meetings.

"Now I know what's important," he kept repeating. "Now I know what's important. I've wasted all of my money in the past. I am thirty-five years old. Now, I know what's important."

I was immediately suspicious of him. I had seen this pattern too many times before with my sister. One minute bragging she was clean, the next minute snorting up the rest of her savings account, years of Christmas and Birthday card money gone within days.

My father swore by his work.

"All right," I finally agreed, and we set up a contract for the first part of the project. What was initially going to take a week turned into a month.

"That's to be expected with home improvement," I told myself, and then hid my two gold rings from my deceased grandmother in the change compartment of my purse before leaving the house.

"You've got a pretty laugh," he said one day when we were alone, scratching his four leaf clover jail tattoo on the side of his neck. *Lucky. Did he think the clover would offer him protection? Would it keep the needle from sliding into his arm again? Would its rare four leaves offer a medicinal cure for his longing?*

Finally, the project was almost complete. There was only a day's work left, so I taped the final payment to the door of the bathroom before I left for work. When I came home, the check was gone, but nothing had been touched inside the bathroom. The tile was scattered around the floor. Only half of the room was painted, and the cut out in the Sheetrock for the mirror cabinet was crooked. We called his cell phone, which had been disconnected. Surprise. Surprise.

Lucky. Lucky him- A naïve wife paid him before the job was finished. *Lucky him-* He has a check big enough for a three-day binge. There is a joke everyone learns at *Nar-Anon*: *How do you know when an addict is lying?* Answer: *When his lips are moving.*

I was mad at myself: I should have listened to my gut. I tried not to think about the money we had lost. At least he had finished installing the new bathtub. I slid down into the comfort of a hot bubble bath. There was one problem. I was too big to fit.

~

Most of the couples were just sitting and listening to the lecture by the board certified anesthesiologist. However, of course, there was *the one*. There always seemed to be *the one* at the classes. She started out by raising her hand and asking why the percentage of epidurals in Maryland was so much higher than in Virginia. She knew the exact percentages and recited them by memory to the anesthesiologist.

The anesthesiologist must have already been through this line of fire with another person before, because he responded without a second of hesitation. He said that the epidural rate tended to be higher in more educated and affluent areas.

The woman continued to question the procedure, spouting off statistics and research like she was defending her dissertation thesis. Everyone in the room started rolling their eyes. The anesthesiologist kept his cool and the woman finally stopped talking, but only after the anesthesiologist had dimmed the lights and directed us with his hands to pick up the packets of information on the side tables.

I wondered if the woman was the same way with her husband, who was sitting silently beside her, his young face expressionless next to her beet red one. Did they debate until he resigned, *I give in. You are right.*

You are right about everything. I sat there, on the fabric covered seat of the folding chair, and wished her a rebel child, one who would want a devil tattoo at age twelve and run away at least three times, causing her to have a nervous breakdown and completely forget about her anti-epidural stance. I wished her a child like my sister, a child who would disagree with her just to disagree, a child just like her.

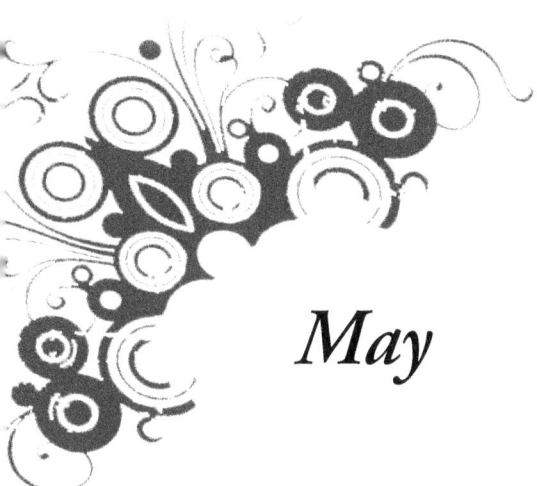

May

Sex was sporadic by the time I reached six months. Some days, I could feel my desire pulsing like a thick rope. All my daily energy was focused in my pelvis, and I could barely stop my hands from gravitating between my thighs. Other days, sex placed second to paying the bills or hiccupping. In addition, there was the added complication of having a third party in the picture.

No one I knew would talk honestly about the problems with sex during pregnancy. My pregnancy books breezed by the topic, stating, "For some women, sex during pregnancy can be a bit awkward. For others, it is an exciting component of the pregnancy." When I asked other pregnant women about it, they just nervously laughed and changed the subject.

My mind wandered as my husband groaned: Could the baby feel it? Could the baby tell the difference between a bump from a forgotten doorknob and the thrust of penetration? Was the baby worried, comforted, or scared by the sudden intrusion so close to his world? It felt too crowded, to have all of us down there. We needed a crossing guard to organize the movements, to keep all of us from running straight into one another, full force and unable to brake, like a runaway train.

~

Half of the stares planted a glowing halo above my head. Grandmothers, little girls, and church-going moms approached me and touched my stomach. My pregnancy automatically propelled me into the sacred category. I was as divine as the angel Moroni, blowing his messenger's horn on the top of the Washington D.C. Mormon temple. I smiled back at the strangers and felt guilty, as if I had taken communion or the Sabbath sacrament after a one-night stand.

For the other half of the people I encountered, my belly had two slick red horns. I was a physical billboard for intercourse, and my swollen breasts were two magnets for groping eyes. I watched the way some women immediately examined my left hand for a wedding ring, hoping not to find one so that they could label a place of shame for me in their inventories. Random men flirted with me. At first, I thought they must not have been aware that I was pregnant. Then, as I was more and more unable to camouflage my stomach, it continued to happen. Were they just being nice, trying to make me feel better about the watermelon that I was lugging around on my waist? Or was it real attraction, my body open and seeded, the path already carved out and waiting?

"Very nice," a man in a complete FILA ensemble winked as I waited in line outside of Checkers. "That's a beautiful thing."

Then, there were the few men who completely denied my existence. They avoided any eye contact as I asked for a price check at Target or a receipt from the Amoco gas station. I was too much like their mothers, unavailable and frightening in my growing state. I could tell that they did not want to think about the pregnancy process at all, as well as their own origins in conception. They still preferred their mothers' answer to their childhood question: *Oh, babies come from the stork, of course. The stork brings them in a white wicker basket, wrapped in soft blankets so they don't catch cold.*

~

The pregnant coworkers were no longer pregnant. They brought their babies in for display, freshly washed and dressed in the latest newborn Baby Gap fashions. I couldn't believe that these women had actually been through the birth process. Their hair was still perfectly in place, and their voices were still confident and strong. I didn't know what I had expected to happen. Perhaps, I thought, two strangers would walk through the door, changed women with different bodies, their cheek muscles pulled tight into their faces. I thought I might see two new wounded women with fresh scars webbed across their skin. No one else seemed shocked that the women still crossed their legs the same way as before, or that their lips moved just as quickly as they did before their children were born.

They took turns passing around their babies and re-telling their *surprisingly easy* labor stories. The babies were adorable, but I was more interested in the women. They were on the other side now; they had already cleared the childbirth hurdle, crossing the line that I was slowly approaching. I asked them an array of questions, like what they were thinking when the babies slid from their bodies, and what it felt like when they first heard the cries of their children. No one could give me a concrete answer.

"I remember a sense of relief," one of the women finally responded, "like a weight was lifted, like I could breathe again."

~

The breastfeeding instructor with the lazy eye brought along a baby doll to help demonstrate the different positions of breastfeeding. She passed it around, and we took turns tilting its plastic head towards our nipples while we awkwardly placed its body in the different feeding positions. It resembled the first day of the gender separated portion of our elementary sex education course, the part where the girls got to pass the feminine hygiene products around the room. I had used the tips of my fingers to touch the maxi pad when it made its way to my desk, and then tried to give it to the girl on my left as quickly as possible. I didn't want the other girls in the class to know that I was already wearing a bloody pad, though it felt like it had to be obvious, the way its existence was burning a hole through my jeans.

We had the same insecure expressions as the doll made its way around the room. The instructor, on the other hand, handled the doll like a real child. She smiled as she brought it to her chest, stroking the plastic cap of yellow hair as she cradled its nude body. Even after the demonstrations were over, she held it to her chest, rubbing its back as she reviewed the top ten reasons to breastfeed.

I pictured her taking the doll to bed with her, placing its open oval mouth to the slit in her old nursing nightgown, comforting its pretend cries in the middle of the night by singing a lullaby. Maybe she was still nursing in her mind, even though her own children were all well past puberty. Maybe this was her way of staying connected to new motherhood, of never having to move on. We all avoided looking at her eyes as we left the classroom, the look of smug students who know nothing of the world and only have a limited amount of time left to ignore it.

~

I had thrown away the first pregnancy journal I started, the journal for the miscarried baby. I didn't want it anywhere around me. It felt like a rotting apple, the first five pages filled out with questions for the baby—*Will you look like Mommy or Daddy? Will you be a boy or a girl?* It went into the trash—along with a half-eaten piece of pizza and an old pair of underwear with broken elastic. I could only imagine where it finally ended up at the dump: at the bottom of a pile of old clogs and used Reynolds Wrap, leaning next to a 1976 issue of *Good Housekeeping*, open to *Jell-O's that Jive* and *Casseroles for the Whole Family*.

After my mother gave me a new pregnancy journal, I immediately shoved it into my pants drawer. I knew that cracking open the blank book would surely jinx the new pregnancy, so I left the book between two pairs of old jeans that I wouldn't be able to squeeze into again for months. I slipped the ultrasound prints underneath the journal and immediately closed the drawer. A few days later, I started feeling guilty thinking about it in the darkness of the dresser, just sitting and waiting for its first entry. I carefully took out the journal. Trying not to bend the binding, I tentatively wrote on the first page. At first, it felt more like fiction, like I was writing to a make-believe child, imagining what it would be like to be pregnant, instead of actually being pregnant.

I taped the ultrasound pictures in—showing the progression from tadpole to mini-baby. Gradually, I found myself able to start documenting the stages. After each writing session, though, I immediately buried the journal back in the middle dresser drawer, covering it with my favorite old pair of faded Levi's.

~

I had been so obsessed with my pregnancy that I had literally forgotten I entered the short story contest until I received an email from the final judge of the Artscape competition, a local English department chairwoman, stating that I was one of the five winners. The winners would all have their stories published in a chapbook, and we were invited to read at the summer festival. I was thrilled and terrified. I loved publishing my work, but I dreaded reading it. I was always self-conscious. By the time I finally relaxed, I was back in my chair, slapping myself inside my head for stuttering and shaking behind the podium.

The reading would be in mid-July, a little over a month before I was due, in one of the lecture halls at the University of Baltimore. I had been to the lecture hall before, fifteen years prior. It was the summer when my high school creative writing teacher had read his winning poetry collection at Artscape. I remembered how professional he seemed, standing up at the veneer podium, describing the process of each poem's development into his chapbook. After he had finished the reading, he had thanked his family and his students and we beamed back from the audience, pleased with our influence on his award.

I tried to imagine myself up there at the podium. Alone, in a balloon sized maternity dress and twelve inch swollen ankles, I knew my breath would cut out first. Then, my hands would start to shake and sweat would begin to drip from under my chin. I would begin to feel dizzy, and the queasy feeling in my stomach would soon increase to intense nausea.

"I'd be delighted to read," I emailed back to the judge of the contest after dinner. She couldn't see my face, grimacing at the thought of what was coming.

~

Due to the unexpected news of the Artscape competition, I suddenly had a burst of creative energy. I decided to write a poem. I hadn't written anything since the short story many weeks before. The pregnancy felt like a monstrous sponge within me, soaking up every bit of excess creativity and impulse.

While I waited for inspiration to kick in, I saw a pop-up ad on Google for a poetry contest judged by Madonna. I clicked on the ad and read the information about the contest. It called for poems about music. The winner would be hand picked by Madonna herself and would win a framed copy of the poem, designed personally by her majesty.

The skeptical part of me knew that it had to be a scam. Madonna didn't have the time to read thousands of bad poems. The best possible scenario was that the reader would be one of Madonna's many assistants, perhaps a tiny man named Oscar, with impeccable clothes and a smoothly shaven head. He would sort through the last round of poems, stamping Madonna's signature on the winning entry. The idealistic part of me knew that her manicured hand was just waiting to click onto my poem. She would barely finish the fifth line before she would be calling her agent, requesting that I write the lyrics to her next ballad.

I remembered the recent *Enquirer* cover that I had perused while standing in line at Safeway. In the top right corner was a snapshot of Madonna and her children, Lourdes and Rocco, strolling through a London park. The headline implied that Madonna wanted to get pregnant again. Our common experience of pregnancy was a sure way to guarantee her attention. I just needed to link *music* to pregnancy for my plan to work.

I was lying in bed, watching my belly move, when the metaphors started to come:

> *The beat is within—*
> *A heart,*
> *tiny like a wet moth*
> *flickers inside me.*
> *The child sings*
> *late at night,*
> *carving songs*
> *into my body*
> *with small hands.*
> *Next to me,*
> *you breathe,*
> *unknowingly,*
> *filtering out the light*
> *like a dark wood,*
> *your body a smooth*
> *casing of sound.*
> *I dream of movement,*

the child
turning to the beat,
my lover
still sleeping
with soft breath.
I nestle back into sleep,
my hands holding
in the rhythms
of my life,
this child,
this moment of music
only we can feel.

She was sure to feel some sisterhood with me. She would read the poem and touch her hand to her flat stomach, remembering her pregnancies and the light taps of her children inside her body. She would smile as she lifted her Prada T-shirt to see a lone microscopic stretch mark barely visible above her left hip. I emailed the poem and checked for a reply everyday. After a week, I only checked every other day. After a month, I only checked once a week. Eventually I had to accept the fate of my little poem, floating out in cyber-space with the rest of the world's unread junk mail.

~

My belly button was starting to pop out, and all of the hidden fuzz and dirt was finally being freed. I thought some of the lint might have been from the orange throw rug I used to hide under when I was scared I would get a spanking from my father. The dirt looked like the red clay from the new well, drilled in the backyard when I was nine.

I looked at the new baby skin rising out at the base of my belly button and wondered if this was how my skin used to look when I was younger, the time when a single scar would stand out on my arm, swollen and red next to the smooth curve of my elbow. Now, injuries just blended right into the growing map of marks on my body.

There was a dark circle forming around my belly button like a planetary ring. It blended into the scar from my belly ring, a crooked mouth that widened with each passing day. Underneath the circle, a black line tracked down my pelvis to the top of my pubic hairline. Lines were also forming around my neck that could pass for dirt necklaces. My mother licked her finger and tried to wipe them off at Sunday dinner, assuming that I had forgotten to wash my neck. I also had little skin flaps growing on my neck and nipples. They were miniature raised moles, the kind that my ninth grade teacher had, the ones I could not stop staring at during our *Treasure Island* class discussions.

My nipples had changed too. They had darkened and widened so much that I looked like one of the tribal women in a *National Geographic* magazine. I could still picture the first photograph of a naked pregnant woman I had ever seen in that magazine. I had stared at the picture when my parents were out of the living room, at the Nigerian woman with long pointed breasts and a huge barreling belly, cooking yams on the fire, her pelvis barely covered by a flap of green cloth. Even then I could tell the woman trusted her body enough to follow the raw experiences of her mothers before her, to accept her instincts instead of her mind. Her body worked within the motions of the world, understanding the dust, the insects, and the trees. She automatically knew what root to rub on a deep cut and what herb would make her dream of her upcoming child.

~

"I've already taken three CPR classes," my husband stated at least twelve times as we drove to the hospital for the CPR course.

"Well, I haven't, and we are supposed to take these classes together," I snapped back. He huffed and puffed. And then all of the doubts started flooding into my mind, making me question how we were ever going to be good parents when we couldn't even make it ten miles without a squabble. I envisioned late night living room fights, a three-year-old crouched under his bed, hands over his ears to drown out the noise.

When we walked into the classroom, I wondered if any of the other couples had been arguing on the way over. Most of the husbands were picking at their nails. The wives were surveying the room, sizing up each other's bellies and the latest maternity outfits. A few husbands massaged their wives' arms, not knowing what else to do, but knowing that keeping their hands busy would keep them out of trouble longer.

Another duo team taught the CPR class. These women also looked like sisters, with their long brown hair, flat chests and tortoise shell glasses. They had their lecture down to a science too, taking turns back and forth without missing a beat. They had even choreographed their bodies so that the one speaking was always standing slightly in front of the other.

First, the instructors played a short film on child safety. It was a horror film. It demonstrated how my home was actually a dungeon of poisons and torture devices. The film depicted a house from a toddler's perspective, beginning with a small boy running straight towards a knife that was hanging off the edge of a kitchen counter. After that narrow escape, the boy reached for the handle of a pot of water boiling on the stove. Next, the toddler tried to stick a fork into a plug outlet and then attempted to drink bleach from the open cabinet under the bathroom sink.

Now I was not only terrified of having this baby, but I was also terrified of my own house. I pictured it down at the bottom of our hill, the weeds growing over the windows like treacherous thorns, lightening ready to strike through the front window at any moment. Maybe there was even an earthquake waiting to happen, a fault line that the realtor conveniently forgot to tell us about.

The instructors pulled out two bright red pointer sticks and stood on either side of the poster taped to the chalkboard. They took turns explaining the directions for proper CPR implementation with an infant:

1. Open airway: Look for movement of the chest and abdomen, Listen for sounds of breathing, Feel for breath on your cheek, Open airway with finger, Remove foreign object if present.

2. Rescue breathing: Position head and chin with both hands, Seal your mouth over mouth and nose, Blow gently, enough air to make the chest rise and fall two times.

3. Feel for pulse: Pulse present, continue one breath every 3 seconds, No pulse, start chest compressions.

4. Chest Compressions: Compress chest ½" to 1", Alternate 5 fast compressions with 1 breath, Compress chest 100 times per minute.

The instructors then stepped out of the room and returned with two dolls. One doll was an infant doll, and the other doll was a five-foot adult. They put plastic protectors in the dolls' mouths and let us know that we would be demonstrating the maneuvers that we had just learned.

I blanked when it was my turn. Was it six breaths, then a push? Was I supposed to check for breath first and then start the presses? How many repetitions did I complete for an adult? I looked at the open mouth of the adult doll, the gaping hole retching up clear plastic protection wrap. I didn't want to put my mouth over it. I wanted to run out of the room. One of the instructors gave me little hints, and somehow I got through the demonstration. She handed me a certificate of CPR readiness, and I thought briefly about hanging it on the wall next to my college diploma.

Luckily, they gave each of us a CPR Steps poster because I couldn't remember a single thing once we left the hospital. I immediately hung the poster up on the refrigerator when we got home. I looked at the black and white sketch on the top left hand side of the poster. It was a sketch of a mother administering CPR to her baby. It looked like a kiss, so easy, like everything does in black and white.

~

This time I was kneeling over our old white claw tub in the dream, carefully draping a warm washcloth over the clot baby's forehead. I didn't know how I had arrived at the spot. I only knew that the water was getting too hot, and I was worried that it would burn the clot baby's raw limbs. I reached for the hot faucet, but then realized it had broken off and there was no way to stop the scalding water from filling the tub. The clot baby was too delicate, and it would surely fall apart if I attempted to lift it from the water.

I could hear people laughing outside of the bathroom, their voices overlapping one another like playing cards. No one cared about what was going on in the bathroom. They were too busy and distracted. I was the only one there for the baby.

The clot baby sunk deeper into the rising water. Its legs were beginning to separate and break off as the tub started to overflow, and I felt the wetness covering my knees. I tried to find the drain, but I couldn't feel the opening underneath the murky water. I kept searching with my fingers, running my hand back and forth over the rough bottom of the tub.

"Don't worry," I cried, as the clot baby's body sunk further down into the water, "I will take care of you."

~

Twenty-eight weeks was the marker, the 60% line, and the point at which the fetus was sometimes able to survive birth. My pregnancy books stressed the complications with the delivery of a baby at this stage: the lungs were not able to breathe on their own yet, the liver was inadequately developed. It was a sketchy existence for a baby at this point, but it *was* an existence.

What would it be like to have my baby at twenty-eight weeks, to run my fingers over my baby's brittle shoulder, touching the hair covering his entire body, so soft and fine that it would make me shutter? I saw my baby in the incubator, his legs like two little pens, and his fingernails too small to see, with only hints of crescents at the tips of his fingers. I would be one of those mothers at the side of a closed incubator, forbidden to touch my child, only allowed to look at the twenty tubes hooked into his body, the oxygen taped like a tiny scuba mask over his face.

Twenty-eight weeks. Twelve weeks early. Three months early. I placed an asterisk on my desk calendar at the twenty eight-week mark. Crossing the solid black line of the day labeled *May 28* was my next goal. I got more nervous the closer I got to it. What if I delivered on *May 27*? What if I got to the 59% line *instead*? I would be so close to a passing "D," but still in the failing category. Would God take pity on me and install a birth curve?

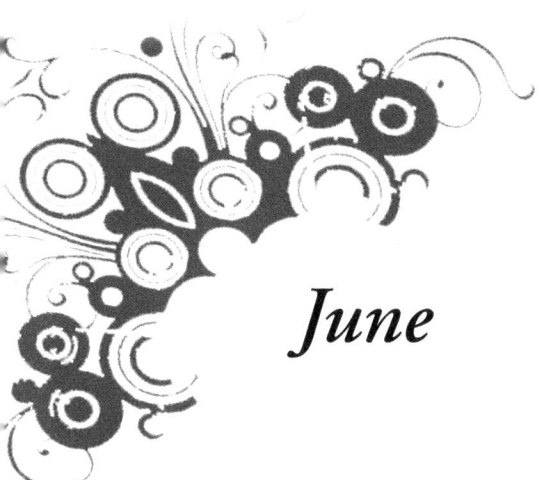

June

My body temperature surged at least ten degrees. I started to feel the pregnancy *heat* that I had heard about from several other women. None of them had mentioned the sour sweat that accompanied it and smelled like rotten onions. I had tried four different types of deodorants without any luck. The scent seemed to thrive on the summer heat.

At first, I thought the house was too hot and dragged an extra fan into the bedroom at night. Without any relief, I turned the window air conditioner unit to MAX and started sleeping naked. I fantasized about panting like one of the dogs, my tongue hanging out of my mouth while the moisture dripped onto the kitchen floor, if that was what it would take to cool me down.

I had never been this hot before. It was a constant heat, a heat that settled in my bones and secreted through my sweat. Every move I made was sticky and uncomfortable. I couldn't get away from the evidence. I saw hot outlines of my hands as they came off the stairway railing. Shadowy spots from my hips remained for hours on the front door screen. Traces of humidity clung to the hair on the bottom of the shower drain, the follicles pulsing from the overload. Even my fingers left steaming prints in the margins of *Moby Dick*, next to the crew's midnight sightings of a silver spout, blowing too far and alluring in the distance to be anything else but their desired whale.

~

My mother called to tell me that my uncle had been assigned to hospice care, and he was given three to six weeks left to live. *Hospice* meant they had given up hope. They would not be resuscitating him. He had graduated to *the dying folder*, the last folder he would ever have in this life. The state hospital had approved his move to Stella Maris, an assisted living and hospice facility, which was only four miles from my parents' house. I drove over to help my mother move his belongings to his new home:

2 black raincoats

5 pairs of grey corduroys with holes in the knees

10 pairs of striped boxer shorts

8 pairs of black socks

15 T-shirts with different amphibian decals

a thin toothed comb

11 Whale Songs CDs

6 Playboy magazines

a crumbling mica rock with his initials, RP, carved into it

a pigeon feather

15 paperclips strung together in a chain

a Blondie-Parallel Lines album cover with no album inside

He was in constant pain now, to the point that he had pulled out the last straggly hairs from his red beard to distract himself from the knives he felt slicing through his brain. He was trying to hurt anyone who came near him, so the doctors had to triple his morphine dose and the nurses cut his long pointed nails down to blunt stubs while he was sleeping. I was afraid to go see his watery eyes, his face eaten away like vulture left overs. I didn't want to see his black and blue arms, the needles jammed into his bruised veins, and the loose hospital socks falling off of his cold feet. I was afraid to see death coming.

I was in my own final category, *Third Trimester*, finally past the twenty-eight week mark. I should have been jumping for joy, organizing the baby's closet, and working on the baby book. Instead, I bit my nails and bought new contact paper for the rusting kitchen shelves. I picked the retro print with the sketches of old blenders and bright oranges. It reminded me of my grandmother, my uncle and my mother's mother. It brought back memories of when I would spend the night at my grandparents' house and my grandmother would squeeze fresh orange juice in the early hours of the morning. The sketches were a flashback to the past, of a time when my grandmother was alive and my uncle lived in her basement, a time that would never return. And when the paper was all cut and sized to the bottom of the shelves, I stepped away and noticed how wrong it was for my kitchen, how it looked new instead of old, and how it was already starting to bubble and peel.

~

I shoved down a banana muffin and a decaf coffee before meeting the elementary school rep for a morning out on the road to recruit new schools for our fundraiser. We went by a few schools in Carroll County and decided to hit Chick-Fil-A for lunch around 12:30. The line was atrocious. I waited patiently behind three businesswomen in matching pastel suits who were debating about who was next in line. The thirteen-year old cashier was ignoring everyone, looking at her three-inch acrylic nails with speckled diamonds as she repeated, "Is that to go?"

The voices tuned out first. Suddenly, the volume was so low that I could barely make out the woman in the pink suit, who was now yelling, "You know I was here first!"

The tunnel started next, a black tube that framed my vision, causing the entire restaurant to feel like it was a mile away, down a long cylinder with tiny people and miniature cash registers like dollhouse accessories. I felt myself dropping, my legs folding underneath me.

Suddenly, a hand magically appeared, and someone was helping me off the floor and into a plastic beige booth. I could tell that my coworker was next to me from her voice, though I couldn't see anything but black spots. A cup found its way to my mouth, and my coworker urged me to drink the fizzy soda. I was so dizzy that I thought I might vomit. I put my head down on the dirty vinyl tabletop and watched the legs of the pastel businesswomen as they walked by, the bags of their Value Meals swinging from their hands like prized school lunches. After the room finally stopped spinning enough for me to stand up without falling, my coworker drove me back to the office, and I called my doctor. He said that it sounded like I was dehydrated. He stressed that I needed to eat and drink every three hours during the rest of the pregnancy.

I couldn't concentrate at work. The dizziness had left me exhausted, so I asked to go home early. The long dark tunnel followed me home. I wrapped myself into a cocoon in my bed. Even *CNN* faded into the distance as I drifted into a claustrophobic sleep.

~

My company classified pregnancy as a short-term disability. At first, I thought it was absurd that pregnancy was considered a disability, but then I found out from the other pregnant women in my swimming class that I had a better monetary maternity leave deal than most of them did at their jobs. The short-term disability would continue to pay me 70% of my salary from the date of my doctor's approval until I returned to work, six to eight weeks after the birth. At least half of the other women at the pool wouldn't receive any pay during their maternity leave, and the other half had to take vacation and sick days. I started filling out the paper work and getting the proper signatures. I had to pretend that I was coming back to work, even though I wasn't planning to return.

"So, do you think you'll take any extra time off?" my officemate asked between sips of her Dunkin Donuts coffee.

"Have you found a daycare provider yet?" questioned the coworker across the hall.

I came up with lies on a daily basis, fabricating possible daycare scenarios and plans to buy an electric pump. I created a daycare mom on my street to help with the constant questions at work.

"Oh, she's wonderful," I told the coworker across the hall. "She has three other children. They study Spanish and sign language and do interpretive dance every other Friday."

"Does she have any other openings?" I heard one of the previously pregnant coworkers ask.

"Oh, no. She isn't taking any other kids. I was only able to secure the spot because my husband's shop always fixes her cars."

"You're so lucky," she replied, and I detected a bit of envy in her voice.

I was amazed at my ability to lie without flinching. I actually started to picture the daycare mom, a hearty Polish woman who smelled like waffles and maple syrup. I could see her salt and pepper bun moving as she took turns pushing children on her backyard swing.

I had to fill in my projected date of return and start summarizing my duties for the temporary worker who would be taking my place while I was on leave. I went crazy with my organization, creating color-coded binders and files with alphabetized five year histories of each account. It took a lot of time and kept me from doing my actual job. There was no way a temp would keep up with my fall kick-offs. I had barely handled them the previous year, and there would be twice as many this coming fall.

"Oh, you'll be fine. It'll be a breeze," I reassured the temp when she came in the next Monday. She had on skin tight black jeans and about twenty earrings running down the cartilage of her left ear.

"It looks like a lot of work," she said, her mouth curling downward.

"It only looks that way," I told her and continued to organize and color code to keep my mind off of really working, off the baby, and my constant anxiety.

I wrote all of my doctor's appointments on my desk calendar with a pink highlighter. The *Moms in Motion* swimming classes decorated every Tuesday and Thursday in yellow marker. I circled my remaining childbirth classes in bright blue ink. Each morning I crossed off another day. There were actual work meetings and conferences, but they all blurred together in my mind. I was too busy concentrating on the little bubbles of movement inside my stomach.

"It should work out fine," I told my nervous manager after a planning session for the activities that needed to be covered during my absence. I walked out of his office without any knowledge of what we had just discussed.

~

One of my books described the movements like the flutters of a butterfly, its thin wings flickering against the skin. It was a beautiful image: a young butterfly inside the body, opening its wings for the first time, practicing quick trials before it actually learned to fly.

The first time I felt a movement I thought it was a spider creeping under my khakis, its sneaky legs nestling beneath my underwear. The second time I thought it was my zipper snagging my skirt at the seam. Each time the feeling only lasted a second, and then it was gone. I couldn't be quite sure that it had ever happened. Then I started to feel a lot of gas bubbles, and I wasn't sure if it was my terrible digestive system or the baby that was causing the ruckus.

The movements usually happened in sets of six or eight clusters, pockets of pressure that caught me off guard. Sometimes they bumped and grinded against the walls of my uterus, like they were trying to break through the lining. Other times they tightened like sailor knots, and I grabbed my side in response. Could it be my appendix or an ulcer erupting? I could never be sure that it was just the baby. I wanted the baby to kick in Morse code, to spell out that he was all right in there. I wanted tiny handprints to appear on my belly so that I could count his fingers and know that there were ten of them. I wanted the movements to make sense. I wanted to understand their choreography and this symphony that was going on inside my body.

~

The cashier handed me the scanning gun, and I was on my way, zapping up my registry at Baby Depot. There were so many products for so many different baby activities that I didn't know where to begin. I brought my mom along to help, but she was as confused as I was.

There were at least forty different types of pacifiers, ten styles of breast pumps, over forty car seats, at least thirty strollers, and a whole wall of different sized and shaped nipples. How was I supposed to know what type of bottle nipples the baby would like? Which car seat would be the most comfortable for a tiny neck? Did I actually need a wipes warmer? Every nightmare story I had ever heard on the news about babies dying from recalled items was running its reel through my mind.

It was a completely different experience from registering for my wedding. I knew we would use the items on the wedding registry. The baby registry was a phony registry. The items I picked seemed arbitrary. I zapped a swing, a high chair, a baby bathtub, and a breast pump. I was going on blind faith that the scanner was leading me in the right direction. First, it pulled me left, then right. I let it lead me all around the store like a divining rod.

"We didn't have any of these things when I had you," my mother kept repeating. "I just bathed you in the sink, used regular towels, and washed your cloth diapers in the washing machine."

It was amazing what good marketing was making me think I had to purchase to be a good mother. I could only imagine what terrible injustice I would be doing to my child if I didn't buy him a bouncy relaxer with a shaded hood and activity bar. Even the names of the products made my mind race: diaper genie, mega-saucer, layette, and onesie. It was another language that I didn't understand yet, one made up of soft syllable words and bubble letters, a language with its own blue and pink rules.

~

The second part of the childbirth classes was a set of three Lamaze sessions. The brochure said not to forget to bring two pillows to the class, and all of our pillows were covered with pet hair and stained with unidentifiable marks, so I ran out before the first class and purchased two Target brand pillows with crisp light blue pillowcases. Sure enough, when we walked into the room that evening, every couple had nice clean pillows with matching cases.

The first class began with an informational lecture. We learned about the different stages of labor with the help of an overhead projector. The instructor was a delivery nurse who had a slight lisp. Her lisp was comforting in a weird way. The nasal ring of her voice made me feel sleepy. She took her wax pencil and pointed to *Transition* on the overhead, the point where we would retreat into ourselves, the point where, as she stated, "You will call your husband an asshole and try to claw out his eyes." We all laughed when she described this scene, but I secretly wondered what the animal inside of me might say at that point.

She explained that the pain and contractions were part of the birth process, and they actually helped the baby to move along the birth canal.

"To have a baby," she repeated throughout the lecture, "you have to have contractions."

Suddenly, the pain and labor seemed linear, instead of just a huge mass of pain waiting to fall on my head. I tried to keep thinking of the process as natural, like the small contractions of my period, like the burn of my calf muscles at aerobics—all needed, all necessary, to achieve the goal. It still terrified me.

The second half of the class involved a practice session on the floor with our pillows and partners. She turned out the lights and had us pretend that we were in stage one of labor. Our goal was to relax, to picture a long beach with a pier that extended into the distance. She told us to walk along the pier and look down at the sand on either side of the salt-worn planks.

As the instructor spoke, her soft lisp started to pull me into a trance, and my belly weight began to lift with the strong details of her visualization exercise.

I was there, at the abandoned beach.

You are now walking off the pier. Your body is as light as the air. As you step into the sand, feel the grains between your toes.

I flexed my feet inside my sandals and followed her cue. My beach grew darker under my lids. I could feel the pillow behind my back, and behind that, my husband's chest moving in and out with his breaths.

You see a little stick there on the sand. Pick it up and start to write your baby's name in the sand, softly and slowly. There is no need to push hard. The stick will sink right in.

I could hear the warm slush of the stick through the sand and felt the slight resistance as the stick started down the long slope of the A.

You are on the next letter. Your stick is now an extension of your finger. The sand is sliding up past your fingernail. The tide comes in and brushes up against your heel.

I felt the lick of the water on my heel. Its dark green tongue almost reached my arch as I drew a D down and around in a half circle.

The sand is warm, and you are perfectly at ease here on this beach, writing your child's name in the sand. Finish writing the name. Feel the sand and the warm sun. Everything is fine here. Everything is safe. Feel the sand parting around your finger. Hear the water cresting in the distance. See your child's name there on the sand. Step back. Feel the slight heat on your back. Step back. See the name. Step back. Open your eyes.

The room was barely visible behind the dark spots that immediately rushed to my eyes. I heard the sea rush away with its lolling sounds, but the feeling of pressing my finger into the sand stayed with me for the rest of the night. It was a very safe sensation, a part of me covered and hidden from the world.

~

I started having throbbing pain in my pelvis, and it was more than just discomfort. I couldn't understand how other pregnant women could still skip and run when I could barely make it off the toilet. It hurt so much that I literally couldn't walk down the steps. I had to turn to my side, grasp the railing, and edge my way down with my knees bent.

The other pregnant women in my swimming class just nodded when I explained why I was walking as fast as a ninety year old.

"I have a lot of pressure too," each one replied, before climbing up the pool ladder without a flinch.

I told my mother about the pain, and she asked me if I thought it could be varicose veins. She had developed them in her labia with each of her pregnancies. When she was pregnant with my younger sister, she could barely stand up by the end of the ninth month. She said that it felt like she had a headache in her crotch, all the blood rushing into the skin, her vaginal folds swelling like purple flippers. I didn't think that I had varicose veins, though I couldn't quite be sure since I couldn't see past my stomach. I felt around down there. There might be some swelling, but I couldn't be sure.

The doctor took a peek at my next visit. "No, you look okay."

"Does this hurt?" he asked, pressing a finger down in the middle of my pelvis.

Pain screamed through my entire lower body. "Yes!"

"It's pelvic symphysis. Your pelvis is separating a little too early. It's due to the hormones." He pulled my gown back together. "It will probably get more painful the closer you get to delivery. You might need to be on bed rest by the end of the pregnancy. I can write you a note to stop working when it's necessary."

The doctor left the room, and I re-dressed. I was actually relieved that it was something concrete, and that I was not imagining the hard block of pain between my legs. I was also relieved that I would be able to get orders to stop working early. It was becoming torturous to walk into the office each morning, my mind completely distanced from the job, my body not far behind in its separateness.

Work, on the other hand, expected me to stay until I went into labor. They wanted every hour that they could get from me: *Oh, the contractions are still ten minutes apart. You can still make some more calls--just one more account, for the team.*

I walked out of the doctor's office with some confidence of knowing at least the direction that this pregnancy was taking me. A janitor moved a little to the left to let me fit into the elevator. I accidentally nudged a teenage girl when I tried to get to the elevator floor panel, but then I stopped when I saw the button of the first floor was already lit bright red.

~

My mother had the list up on the refrigerator at her next Sunday dinner, next to the copy of the ultrasound picture that I enlarged for her at the office on our fancy new copier. The list was in the same spot where I used to hang my report card, highlighting every *A* with a yellow marker and leaving the annoying *B*'s unnoticed in the beige background.

My ultrasound looked like a fake print next to the numbered list of hospice rules. The baby's profile was only a computer-based suggestion; a representation of a baby that I still questioned was even there. The hospice rules list was definite, the letters dark and clear from an alphabet that had been established for centuries. The list was reality, proof of my uncle's upcoming end, his soon-to-be cease of existence:

1. *The patient's comfort is the most important factor*
2. *Allow the patient as much movement and independence as is appropriate.*
3. *Do not dwell on the illness, but allow the patient to talk about it if he/she wants.*
4. *Give the patient respect even when he/she needs assistance with very personal tasks.*
5. *Find out the patient's preference for final arrangements.*
6. *There is no diet for patients. He/she should eat whatever he/she wants.*
7. *Pain management is very appropriate and needed.*
8. *Do not call 911.*
9. *Do not try to resuscitate the patient.*
10. *Learn the signs of the end.*

I wondered what the signs of the end were: Seeing a faint white light at the end of a narrowing tunnel? Speaking in tongues? Feeling the heart gradually slow to a still? Or, was it the soul beginning to separate from the body, the desire to live breaking from the prison of the flesh and moving out into the freedom of the air?

~

My husband ordered a family sized baby pool from *Amazon.com*. He said it was to help me relax, though he was the first one to slide under its prickly cold surface after it arrived. I climbed into my whale-sized bathing suit and carefully waded in. The water was freezing. The *just out of the hose* chill ran through my body, and I felt a little cold for the first time in weeks.

We hung out in the pool for over an hour while the clouds hurried past the sun. I turned over onto my belly and let the water hold up my weight as I pulled my body back and forth with my arms to create a small current. My body was a kaleidoscope. Inside, colors swirled into patterns, thousands of angles and lines constantly moving into the next formation. Outside, I was a plain brown tube, a barrel of puffy skin. It hurt to climb out of the pool. It hurt to do anything.

During the next few days, I watched the pool grow a stagnant film across its surface. Bugs started to collect along the rim and hard black shells filled the bottom, mixed with twigs and seedpods. The flat blue bottom began to turn a milky green. Underneath the pool, the grass started to die. I didn't care. The pool was outside, and nothing outside mattered to me anymore.

July

I wore the same brown dress with the circus tent waist that I had been wearing everyday since June to the Artscape reading. Of course, it was over 100 degrees that day, and so humid that everyone who walked by me at the Lutherville light rail station stared and said, "You must be miserable!" After five sluggish minutes on the light *snail*, I noticed an unpleasant odor and realized that it was coming from my armpits. I looked down at my story, to distract myself from the smell and my anxiety, which was growing by the second. I still hadn't re-read the story since I had received the email notification about the winning entries. Once upon a time, I had practiced for hours before a reading, repeating my poems until I knew them by heart. I would read them in front of the mirror, first from the left profile, then from the right. Today, the audience was lucky that I had shaved up to my mid-calf.

The *light snail* was so slow that I ended up rushing into the lecture hall ten minutes late, just in time to hear the judge call my name from the podium and look around to see if I was in the audience. I wobbled down the aisle, feeling hundreds of eyes on me as I approached the podium. The stares immediately began to cause a blockage in my air pipe, and I struggled for breath as I stumbled through the first paragraph:

Halfway. She pictures the word like the precise step of a tightrope walker, his bare arms slick with sweat, balanced in a straight line above the hushed crowd. Halfway across and halfway on the rope, he pauses, lets his eyes linger towards the audience, then starts to lose his balance. She smiles as he falters, grabbing for the air.

I looked up to see my sister coming in late, asking a man in the back row to move his legs so she could get to the seat next to my mother.

This is what she pictures as halfway, not the peeling wall she continues to flake away next to her single bed, or the empty bed across the room, the stained gray mattress blank of any knowledge of its last resident, this time, relapsed in only a week. The word does not even sound like the noises she begins to hear, the six other women in the house, already starting to stir, all required to attend two meetings a day.

After the microphone echoed my quivering voice enough for the audience to know that I was a complete nervous wreck, I finished the second paragraph and gained a small ounce of composure.

Half-awake, she tries to push off her covers, to walk to the end of the long hall to the bathroom, but the water is already being turned on, someone else's hand is testing the temperature before parting the curtain and stepping in. So she decides to stay perfectly still, to let the numbness of sleep give her a few more minutes of comfort. Soon, that will not be enough, and a cigarette will hold its own claim halfway in her mouth.

The shower stops and still she does not move, watching the morning light attempt to break through the star shaped rip at the bottom of the shade.

She wants to take her finger and rip the hole open wide enough to fit her fist through. She laughs as she sees her whole arm going through the hole, then the window, waving in a bloodied blur to the old woman across Linwood, the one who is always staring out of her window with a sneer, pulling her green curtain across her sagging chest like a shield.

The words started to gradually become words again, not the little daggers that they had been at the beginning of the reading. The story grabbed back its tangible scope, and the consonants began to blend into one another, instead of ripping my tongue with their prickly legs.

She misses the Coke can and drops the ashes onto the carpet as she finally moves one leg out into the air. The room's cold chill still startles her after two months. Her leg hair bristles with goose bumps. She stumbles across the room before she hears the hum of the shower start again.

A little more time, and she curls up next to her closed door, wrapping a nearby pair of crumpled jeans around her cold legs. With her head against the wood door, she can hear the coffee maker burping its last few drops downstairs. Someone slams the screen door and heads to the bus stop.

By the time I made it to the last paragraph, I wondered what all the fuss was about inside my brain.

She puts her cigarette out on the door and watches the ashes immediately whiten like an old mold. She takes her pinkie finger and wipes the warm ash off. Nothing. There is not even a sign or splinter that she is here now, just the old door and the residue on her own skin. She does not think she will be able to get back up. Her jeans are rooting around her thin legs. She can barely balance her head without feeling nauseous. Even her fingers are uneven, nine clammy, one small one gray with ash. And that is what bothers her the most today, her fingers, and their surprising weight.

Afterwards, my family reassured me that I didn't look a bit nervous, which meant I must have looked like I was going to have a stroke. The judge handed out the chapbooks, and I was thrilled to see that my story was the first selection in the chapbook. For a moment, I forgot that I was pregnant, and turned to start the post reading celebratory chatter, but then I felt a sharp pain ripping through my pelvis and knew I would be heading home.

~

"Labor is now getting into full swing," the instructor of our second Lamaze class at the hospital explained. "You won't be pushing yet, just concentrating on the contractions. Three shallow breaths and one blow. Quietly pronounce *hee, hee, hee, who*. Try it with me." She pulled her mouth back to reveal a set of cigarette stained teeth.

I tried to concentrate and to follow her instructions, but in my mind I was actually down the hall from the class, looking for the nursery window. I had on a pink robe with little blue butterflies, and pink fuzzy slippers to match. My labor had been *surprisingly easy*. I wasn't feeling any pain as I placed my palm against the clear window and saw a little pink and blue striped hat in the portable crib, with two full lips underneath, nestled into a sound sleep.

"Now repeat," the instructor directed, "*hee, hee, hee, who.*" The nursery curtains quickly shut, and I opened my mouth to join the rest of the hissing around me.

After a ten-minute break, we met at the ob admitting area for a tour. I sucked in every detail: the peach color of the walls in the waiting room, the dark wood of the receptionist's desk, the soft click of the released lock as the instructor scanned her card to open the double doors to the delivery area.

My husband and I stayed to the back of the tour, watching the other couples in front of us pause to check out the admitting/waiting area before moving on. Everyone was quiet as we walked past three pre-surgical prep rooms that the instructor explained were only for Cesarean sections. I recognized the light yellows of the wildflower print on the wall of the last room as we walked by it. It was the same room where I had waited for my D & C a few months before.

"Hopefully, you won't need to be in *there*," she whispered, pointing to the surgery room door at the end of the hall like it was the entrance to hell.

"I think that was where I was before," I said to my husband.

"Was that the room?" he said, not requiring a reply.

I suddenly felt a strange sense of injustice, in that I had already seen this part of the tour. I wanted to stop the tour to notify all of the other couples that I had already been there, in the faded gray hospital gown, in the waiting room, and then strapped down onto the cold silver table of the operating room. Instead, I kept my mouth shut and kept up the tail end of the tour.

We inspected a delivery room next. The hospital had recently remodeled the delivery rooms, and the couples took turns sticking their heads in and responding with the same "Ahhh!" sound. The room had a finished pine floor, with dark maroon walls and hunter green and beige trim. A cherry stained entertainment center displayed a large television above two drawers, and a small sofa seat lined the space under the window. In the middle of the room was the delivery bed, looking out of place from the rest of the domestic décor. Over in the corner a tiny portable crib waited, the overhanging lights turned off, so that I could just make out a blue nasal aspirator resting on the top of the thin white mattress cover. It was hard to imagine that a doctor would soon be placing a baby onto this mattress. It seemed impossible that a baby could actually start to breathe on its own on this mattress—that all it took was a flat surface and a clean sheet to create his first home away from his mother's belly.

The next stop in the tour was the recovery room. That was where we would go after the delivery for the remainder of our stay—two to three days if we had a vaginal delivery and four to five days if we had a c-section. The room was the size of a closet, with barely enough room to walk around the hospital bed. There was a stiff orange vinyl chair in the corner, a sink in the wall next to the bed, and a tiny bathroom in the back that was the size of an airplane stall.

"The hospital is going to remodel these rooms, but they won't be finished until next year," the instructor frowned. "For your *next* delivery," she perked back up, "you'll have a remodeled recovery room."

The nursery was the last stop. All of the women, including myself, ran to the window like it was the monkey cage at the zoo. Noses pressed against the glass, our breath fogged up the pane as we watched the two nurses on the other side. They were talking while they were giving one of the newborns a sponge bath. The baby had on a diaper that was so small it was barely there at all. It was taped around the baby's waist, and its skinny legs dangled down underneath like loose spools. Even though I couldn't hear a word that the nurses were saying, their smiles signaled that something was funny in their conversation.

"Most mothers prefer to keep their babies in their rooms now. The nursery is not what it used to be," the instructor informed us from behind.

It certainly was not the nursery of the movies and television, where babies lined the room while their families peeked in, trying to distinguish one blue knit cap from another. In fact, the knit caps were all yellow in this nursery, so that I couldn't tell which baby was a boy and which one was a girl.

The nursery was also smaller than I had pictured it, with room for only five portable cribs at the most. The walls were white, without any decorations, and the tile on the floor was the same hunter green as the trim in the delivery room. The green seemed too adult for a nursery, too fabricated, like paneling, or stucco.

Then again, nothing could have lived up to the picture I had envisioned of the nursery where my child would be cared for during his first hours. Nothing short of a life size *Fisher Price* Tree house with bassinets swinging from its branches would have impressed me. I wanted to see blue gingham sheets tucked into wicker bassinets, the tips of newborn noses peeking out into the crisp air. I wanted to know a brigade of nurses was getting ready to march in with their starched white uniforms and stiff white hats, armed with warm milk bottles and hand-knitted mitts.

The real life nursery was small and plain. "We keep the curtains closed now for security reasons," the instructor whispered, as if she had just exposed a national secret. "I had to call ahead to get them opened up for us."

~

There was a knock at the door, and I knew who it was as soon as I saw the dark blue suits with the black and white nametags.

"Sister Anderson?" they asked, before the door was barely open.

"I didn't change my last name," I informed the Mormon missionaries through our screen door.

They looked at each other, puzzled by my response. I was still on the *Inactive* missionary visitation list. This meant that for the rest of my life the missionaries would be knocking at my door, pretending that they were just stopping by to remind me of the upcoming church events, never acknowledging the big "I" next to my name on their calling lists.

I used to hide from the missionaries, turning off the lights and running into the bathroom when I saw their rented Ford Escort pull into the driveway. But as I got older, the missionaries started to look more like little boys, like the nineteen-year-old kids that they were, and I gradually stopped the charade.

I knew that they were not supposed to be in a house alone with a woman, so I talked to them through the screen, my huge belly starting to stretch the front panels of my robe apart. I pictured my robe accidentally flying open with a sudden gust of wind; my swollen breasts dangling like cantaloupes above my stomach. Would they shield their eyes and instantly turn away, their pupils dilating in terror? Or, would they peek before wincing at my shaggy pubic hair stretched into the bottom curve of my stomach? Would their god make my body invisible to them; creating a shield of crystalline light that would block their virgin eyes from the sight? I ran through the possible scenarios in my head as they offered their services to help with the lawn.

"I'll check with my husband," I told the taller of the two, the cuter one with the striking blue eyes.

"Just give us a call," he responded, flashing his business card, with the title, *Elder Williams, Missionary, The Church of Jesus Christ of Latter Day Saints.*

"I'll let him know," I reinforced, already fully aware that my husband wouldn't be calling him back.

They left, and the dogs didn't stop barking until the Escort was completely out of the driveway. I thought about the cute one with the blue eyes for longer than I should have. I wondered what his muscles would feel like under the warm sleeve of his temple garment.

~

I started packing. It was a not unlike packing for vacation, but this time the flier that I had received from the last Lamaze class recommended bringing maxi pads instead of a swimming suit. I went over my list repeatedly, comparing it to the ones in my pregnancy books to make sure that I had not forgotten a single item:

- *nursing pajamas*
- *face soap*
- *toothbrush*
- *toothpaste*
- *brush*
- *shampoo*
- *conditioner*
- *ponytail holder*
- *baby outfit to go home in*
- *socks*
- *baby book (place marked for hand and foot prints)*
- *pen*
- *watch for timing contractions*
- *nursing bras*
- *underwear*
- *outfit for me to wear home (big size)*
- *pads*
- *camera (battery charged)*
- *diapers*
- *cap for baby*
- *booties and mitts for baby*
- *car seat- needs to be installed and checked*
- *Moby Dick*
- *this journal*

Still, I kept feeling like something was missing, something more vital and important than toothpaste. I couldn't think of anything else that I might need to bring, yet I still had a small knot in my gut. Maybe I was only forgetting myself, the woman I left back in one of the fast food restaurant bathroom stalls, the line of the pregnancy test still darkening in the sweaty cup of her palm.

~

My weight ballooned to 200 pounds. I couldn't fit into my cute maternity clothes anymore. I was stuck with my husband's XL undershirts and boxers. My legs and ankles were swollen with fluid, and my stomach stretched ahead of me by at least a foot. Even my double chin had a double chin. I didn't recognize myself when I looked in the mirror—there was only an obese woman staring back at me.

When I was lying down, my stomach divided and folded over both sides of my body. It covered my hips like the heavy x-ray apron at the dentist's office. It was hard to accept that this was my stomach. I kept thinking of it as luggage, as the run-down leather suitcase left at baggage claim, going around, and around, and around the terminal.

The stretch marks started to multiply. I initially thought I was in the clear, almost through the eighth month of pregnancy without any sign of one. Then I noticed a small line above my right hip, and literally, overnight, the marks bred like gremlins until purple rips covered my abdomen.

The doctor, thank goodness, didn't say anything about my weight at my next appointment. He did mention the fluid, and I saw him flinch when his finger pressed, literally, into the skin around my ankle. I told myself that it was all fluid gain. It definitely couldn't be the two bowls of ice cream that I was polishing off every night.

I told the doctor that I thought I felt the baby's head under my ribs.

"I don't think it's the head," the doctor said, as he held his hand over the hard lump. "But we'll check next time, when it's closer."

The bulge pulsed back when I pressed on it during the drive home. I couldn't tell what it might be. It could have been the hoof of a horse, a smooth rock, or a tiny globe rotating inside my body.

~

The pelvic pain increased by the day. I could barely make it down the steps to take a shower each morning. Nights were terrible. Every time I rolled over, I felt like there was a stick poking me in my pelvis. It hurt to stand up, to sit, and to walk. I looked at the calendar, down at my swollen feet, back at the calendar, and called my doctor to ask if he could write the okay for me to stop working.

At our morning meeting, I announced to my boss and my coworkers that my doctor was giving strict orders that I shouldn't work past the upcoming Friday. My manager just nodded. After the meeting, I walked by his office and saw his head resting on his desk.

The doctor faxed over my official diagnosis of *pelvic symphysis,* and I was on my way to official disability. I started to clear my desk of any personal items when no one was looking.

"Would you like to continue working from home during these last couple of weeks?" my manager asked.

"I don't think so." I tried not to laugh out loud.

I managed to make it to Friday somehow and was amazed that the events of my last day were normal. Everyone went about their merry way—working, making calls, organizing and filing.

"Call if you need anything," the receptionist said, as I pushed open the front door at the end of the day.

"Sure. Thanks." I paused, waiting for streamers or confetti.

"Good luck," another coworker yelled up front before disappearing back into her cubicle.

"I'll talk to you all soon," I smiled, looking back to see if my surprise cake was waiting in the wings.

"Not too many soap operas!" the receptionist laughed as the door closed behind me.

That was it. I wouldn't be coming back through that door again until I was a mother. I was surprised that the drive home looked the same as it always did. There was the same junk mail in the mailbox that I found there every evening, and the same puddle spot left by one of the dogs near the refrigerator. I pressed the blinking message on the answering machine and heard my husband's voice explaining that he wouldn't be home until around seven o'clock. I sat down on the couch and watched the weather channel, which predicted another week of record heat. The constant noise from the television didn't camouflage the stillness of the house. The dogs were even motionless, their heads sagging on the carpet like old shoes.

~

The *Signs of the End* pamphlet was up on the refrigerator at my parents' house, clipped directly on top of the *Hospice Rules* list. The cover of the pamphlet didn't have any words on it, only the black silhouette of two people, their heads resting on each other's shoulders, their shadows blending into one dark body. It was a subtle and appropriate cover, with no hint of the true content inside. The type set was a delicate font, with words that looked as harmless as wildflowers. It even used the term "loved one," instead of "patient" or "dying person." Its attempts at softness seemed pathetic, as there was no real way to sugar coat death:

> *1. The loved one's extremities may become cool and the color of the skin may darken.*
> *2. There may be an increase in the loved one's sleep.*
> *3. The loved one may experience a pronounced disorientation and confusion of place, time, and people.*
> *4. There may be a decrease of the loved one's urine output with onset of incontinence.*
> *5. You may hear congestion and loud gurgling sounds like marbles rolling around in the chest of the loved one.*
> *6. The loved one may exhibit restless and repetitive movements.*
> *7. There may be a decrease of the loved one's fluid and food intake.*
> *8. The loved one may experience irregular breathing patterns.*
> *9. The loved one may withdraw and become unresponsive to others.*
> *10. The loved one may see visions of people who have already died or places not ever seen during their lifetime.*

I wondered if my uncle could be having visions of his mother, my grandmother, who had passed away fifteen years before. Was she still the same age as when she had died, her hair pinned up into a silver bun with three silver bobby pins, her back pulled over into the hump of scoliosis? Or, was she the mother he remembered from his youth, before his illness took over, a serious brunette with long curls and horn-rimmed glasses?

Would she meet him at the beginning of his journey to the other side, or would he have to search to find her, past lines of other people waiting for their own relatives, crowded and impatient like an airport boarding gate?

I hoped he would finally find the place that he had looked for his entire life, a place where he could live by his own rules, with rivers and caves nestled next to one another like siblings. It would be a place without expectations, where there was no *normal*, where he could finally be at home.

~

"I have heard everything during the transition stage," the delivery nurse told us during our last childbirth class. "Husbands, don't be alarmed if your wives tell you they hate you during this stage. I've seen wives hit their husbands and tell them to get the hell out of the room. They have no way to predict what they'll do at this stage."

"First, ladies," she slowed and lowered her voice; "You will go within, to a place inside your body, trying to escape from the pain." She paused, and we tilted our ears a little closer towards her. It seemed to get darker in the room. "It's your body's natural instinct: to flee from danger," she informed us, and explained the process of transition, of the final moments before our bodies would break apart into two separate beings.

Transition sounded like a P.O.W. camp, like a dark jungle inside my body, hiding a bamboo cage so small I would have to sit cross-legged to fit inside. I could feel the humidity in the cage, the lack of protection from the black bugs that would leave welts all over the body. It was a place hidden from the sun, from any other human being, with only the air whipping through the rough shoots of the cage. It was a place without hope, a place of total despair and no way out.

The husbands looked at each other from across the room. There was true fear in their eyes—a look of panic that the wives pretended not to see. Each husband was wondering what his wife would become. *Would fangs break through her gums? Would she sprout hair from her shoulders and start to growl? Would green venom begin to drool from her mouth?*

The instructor noticed the silence and tried to deflate the transition discussion by making a joke about the upcoming practice session on labor positions. "Remember," she stressed, "no real pushing. We don't need to have any babies born here tonight."

It was our last class, and when it was over and we pulled out of the parking lot, I was a little sad. I was on my own now. There would be no more packets, or sign-in sheets, or new pillowcases without stains or wrinkles.

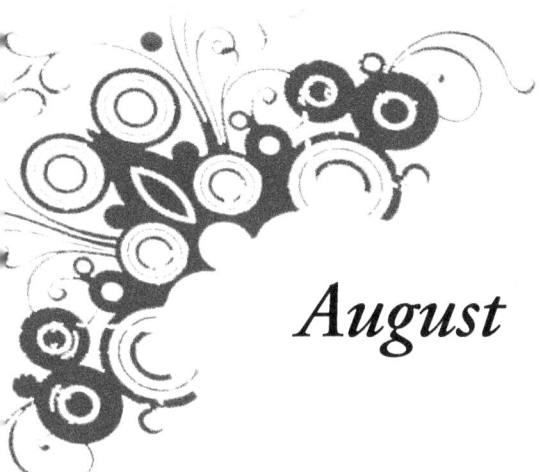

August

My mother's living room smelled of baby powder and clean towels. I sat in the rocking chair in the corner and opened up presents for what seemed like hours. I took my time peeling off the tape, then unfolded and refolded the wraps like fragile fabrics. I held each little washcloth and tube of *Desitin* up for everyone to see, each little bootie a reinforcement that the coming birth might be real, that my child might actually need these clothes, diapers and ointments. I kept looking at my stomach to make sure that it had not disappeared since my last glance, which seemed ironic since my belly was the focus of the celebration.

After I opened all of the presents, everyone congregated around the food table. My mother had made watermelon fruit salad, carving the bottom half of the watermelon rind into a small basket. Honeydew and watermelon balls rested comfortably inside the basket like Easter eggs. Everything at the party was small: the gifts, the food, the favors. Even the guests' clothes seemed to be repelling in the glaring pressure of the summer heat. Tank tops slid off tan shoulders, and my own bra straps refused to stay on my arms.

Before I knew it, people were already starting to leave, and the blur of wrapping paper and fluffy bows was ending. I picked up a little blue sleeper from the top of the gift pile and held it away from my body. It was too tiny to contain a human. It was a doll's outfit, for a plastic doll with a head that nuzzled into my shoulder when I pulled the string screwed into its hollow back.

~

The next day my mother's living room smelled of cardboard and salt. My uncle had died the previous evening. My mother got the call an hour after my shower had ended and arrived at the hospice center within minutes of his passing.

"He just looked like he was sleeping," she explained to us as we ate leftovers from the shower for lunch. She had been the interpreter for his life, the only person who remained with him throughout the years.

One of my uncle's caseworkers called to offer her sympathies. We could hear the conversation from the den. My sister, who had stopped by for free lunch and laundry, pretended to be looking for a better show on the television as she flipped the remote through all of the channels. I picked up a week old newspaper and pretended to work on the word scramble. My father was in the bathroom, humming and flipping through a magazine. My mother was choking up as she thanked the caseworker for her dedication to my uncle over the past few years, for helping to see past his mental illness and his frightening appearance.

My sister asked me if I wanted to watch *Oprah*.

"Sure," I said, since there wasn't anything else to say.

My mother hung up the phone, and my father flushed and came out of the bathroom. My mother wiped her eyes.

"The caseworker said he lived on the outside of his body," she repeated. "She said he wasn't gray like the rest of us. He wasn't afraid to expose his soul, to let his internal creatures meet the rest of the world."

I tried to picture my own internal soul, caterpillars crawling up and down my spine, a praying mantis settled deep inside my liver. I couldn't imagine my soul turning inside out, or my worry hanging loose like drying laundry. Yet, maybe it would be better, to let my barnacles of fear attach somewhere else-- to a tree, to a flagpole, or to the welcome sign hanging from my mother's front door.

My sister flipped the channel to the local news.

"Do you want to watch this instead?" she said.

"Sure," I replied, and returned to my word scramble: A E T D H.

~

At my next appointment I warned the doctor that my pelvic pain had been increasing, but I don't think he really understood until he put one gloved finger inside of me, and I screamed and grabbed the side of the examining table.

"It hurts that badly?" he asked.

"Yes!" I hissed.

"You can take Tylenol for the pain," he suggested, like it was a headache.

I braced myself again for the pain and clenched my jaw as he checked for dilation.

"You are about one centimeter," he said, slapping off the glove and stepping away from the table. "Don't worry, though, some women are at one centimeter for over a month before they deliver."

"Let me check the position now," he said and began pressing his hands against my belly. The hard ball was still up near my ribs, and I waited for him to get around to it.

"This baby is breech," he announced, looking surprised. "Did it turn since the last exam?"

"No, it has been like that the *whole time*," I informed him, emphasizing *whole time* so that he'd know I had been right all along, and he might as well hand over his medical degree to me right then.

"Well, you've still got a couple of weeks. The baby could still turn, but I only want to give it another week. We can try to turn it then, or schedule a c-section if you prefer."

"What do you recommend?" I asked, well aware of his answer.

"I recommend scheduling. We aren't always successful with turning."

"Okay," I said, more calmly than I expected to hear myself sound. I had rehearsed the conversation in my mind since the last appointment.

"Let's see where things stand next week, and then we'll go from there. Oh, and don't be alarmed if you have some spotting today." He headed out of the room. I dressed, and then stamped my parking garage ticket in the usual routine as I left the office.

I drove straight to my parents' house after the exam. My mother was the only one home.

"I've got news," I said with a serious face.

"What is it?" she asked, alarmed.

"The baby is breech, and if it doesn't turn by next week, I'm going to have to have a c-section."

"Okay." She seemed to be saying the words to herself, a bit of pressure released from her eyes.

C-Section. It was one of those things like getting glasses, a speeding ticket, or jury duty. It was someone else's problem. I visualized the long white scar running down the middle of my mother's best friend's stomach. As a child I had imagined the scene of her strapped to the operating table, skin peeled open and pinned to the sides like a biology dissection, as the doctor scooped out her first daughter.

"C-sections are very common now," I informed my mother. "Almost one in three births in the United States are by caesarean," I recited from the latest chapter of my pregnancy book.

"But it still might turn. I've got a week." I knew the baby wouldn't turn. I was already repacking my bag in my head to include a couple more bras and pajama sets. My mother started cooking spaghetti, and I went to the bathroom. There was a faint spot of blood in my underwear. However, this time my heart didn't completely drop into my feet, only to my stomach.

"He told me this might happen," I said aloud to myself.

I called anyway.

"How much spotting should occur after an internal exam?" I asked the nurse. "I'm in my ninth month."

"Not too much," the nurse answered. "It shouldn't last more than twenty four hours or so." It was twenty-two-and-a-half-hours, and I was about to call the doctor again when it finally stopped.

~

I kept the *Signs of Labor* list under my pillow, within inches of my arm, in case I needed to grab it in the middle of the night. I didn't want a single symptom to go unnoticed, to slip into my body while I was sleeping, temporarily unaware of the baby's arrival intentions.

1. *Your bag of waters may rupture.*
2. *Labor contractions may increase in frequency.*
3. *There is not any relief from contractions by a change in position.*
4. *Labor contractions may increase in strength.*
5. *Pain may begin in your lower back.*
6. *Pain may spread to your lower abdomen.*
7. *The pain may spread to your legs.*
8. *Gastrointestinal upset may begin.*
9. *Diarrhea may begin.*
10. *You may experience a discharge that is pinkish and blood-streaked.*

The list was my set of cliff notes, my safety net of clues. I re-read the signs each night just before bed, keeping the answers fresh in my mind like I used to with my high school exam notes, giving them one more glance, and then placing them under my pillow to let the words rise up through the cotton stuffing before settling into my brain.

~

Once I was home on official bed rest, I learned the entire daytime cable television schedule, especially the shows geared towards women.

The Learning Channel was a particular tearjerker buffet. From noon to one o'clock, I watched *A Dating Story*, which followed different couples through nights of planned romance and trendy restaurants. After that, there was *A Wedding Story*. I especially like the Australian weddings, taking place in backyards, barns, and dusty halls. Young buck-toothed grooms grinned while their brides stuffed themselves into frilly homemade dresses.

A Baby Story was on next, a full hour of pregnancy stories and baby deliveries. I usually couldn't make it past the first fifteen minutes without crying. I was amazed at how the women grunted and groaned while the camera rolled and their entire extended family watched in anticipation. I usually had to turn the channel before the actual births happened, my anxiety kicking into full gear, as I did not know which route my delivery story would take. Unlike the one hour episodes, I didn't have my happy ending yet.

And then there was *Lifetime*. *Lifetime* always had great 1980's movie marathons on in the late afternoons. They were completely predictable mysteries with Stephanie Powers and Judith Light in tight sequined gowns. I loved seeing the outdated hair sprayed bangs and long plastic earrings, the business power suits with thin Fava pumps, and the slick black and gold furniture of their beachfront condominiums.

The titles of the movies were classic: *Nighttime Caller, She was Marked for Murder, Deadly Lies*. The mystery was always unraveled at the end of each movie, the bad guy (who usually turned out to be the husband) always exposed for the crook that he was. The beautiful wife, after two hours of worrying and crying, usually found herself in the arms of her young charming attorney.

I wasn't interested in the predictable plots. I couldn't keep my eyes off the women's blue mascara coated eyes and the dangle of the diamond necklaces around their necks. They couldn't possibly be real. They couldn't ever wake up with bad breath, or suffer from a terrible bout of constipation. They surely wouldn't ever pluck new witch whiskers off their chins, and then place them directly on the white rim of the bathroom sink.

~

I could have been scheduling a haircut.

"Would Monday or Thursday work better?" the doctor asked.

"Let's go for Thursday," I replied, knowing that my mother had already scheduled my late uncle's tribute for Wednesday at the state hospital.

"Okay. Thursday at 9:00," the doctor said, as he scribbled down the information on his notepad and started to walk out of the room.

"Wait," I called after him. "What do I need to do?"

"Oh, the nurse up front will let you know everything," he replied and continued down the hall.

"Okay," I stuttered, expecting him to turn around and say, "Just kidding. Here's your caesarean rulebook and guidelines."

He knocked on the second door down the hall, and I heard, "Hi, Mrs. Dobbs, how have you been feeling since your fibroid surgery?" through the wall.

I asked the nurse at the receptionist desk what I needed to know before my c-section the following Thursday.

"Just arrive a half hour early and don't eat or drink anything after midnight," she smiled.

"That's it?" I questioned.

"That's it, hon," she winked. "Good luck."

"Thanks," I mumbled and walked out into the fluorescent glare of the lobby. I had been given more prep instructions for the ultrasounds than I did for this upcoming birth.

Thursday at 9:00.

Thursday, August 23.

I said the date over and over in my head as I rode the elevator down to the lobby.

August 23.

That would be the birthday of my child.

August 23.

~

I didn't think that the pregnancy could feel any more stifling, but the last week proved me wrong. The heat wave continued, and my pelvis constantly ached. I stayed inside in my underwear. I couldn't focus on anything. I couldn't read a single paragraph of *Moby Dick* without losing my train of thought. As soon as I finished a sentence I linked the events to my pregnancy, and the next thing I knew Captain Ahab was pacing outside of a delivery room, checking his watch every other minute and banging his ivory leg against the soda machines.

The only thing I really had a desire to do was to buy baby clothes, so I suffered through the pelvic pain and wobbled out to Hecht's, hunting through the clearance racks for a "find." It felt like I was on a treasure hunt, prepared with the necessary clues: a possible sex (male), a due date (August 23), and the knowledge that this child would probably be at least average size. I ruled out the wrong season, the wrong color, and the wrong price.

Finding the right baby outfit gave me a sense of logic. The outfits were tangible, products at the end of a complicated equation. Six buttons on the front of the shirt, snaps around the crotch, and a giraffe on the pocket saying "It's playtime" in red letters put me at ease. I touched each button and noted the cotton blend, still clean and wrinkle free. I held the outfit I finally picked out in my left arm and paid for it with my right hand. When I got home, I immediately hung it up in the baby's closet. It felt like feathers as I swung it, just a bit, back and forth from the tiny white hanger.

~

We finally cut loose from the backed up State Fair traffic, the mini vans piled high with cheap stuffed animals, glow in the dark necklaces and sticky children, and yielded onto Route 70 to head west to the state hospital for my late uncle's tribute. It wasn't going to be a traditional funeral, as my uncle had elected to have his body donated to science. I didn't want to think about what *science* would do to his brain, extracted from his lifeless body, a mind that had continued to kick and scream like a child pulled away from his mother. Would they find an answer to his years of suffering by coming across a crisscrossed wire? Or, would they discover a pocket of angry nerves finally settled into an exhausted heap?

We entered the hospital and a guard at the front desk filled us in on the correct route to get to the second floor. We took the elevator and walked down several hallways until we got to the right room. The room for the memorial was completely empty except for a clear plastic display which included my uncle's name and the childhood photographs that my mother had collected. They were pictures of a freckled boy just waiting for puberty to arrive, with no way to know what it would actually bring. There was no hint that his lengthening body would begin to break out into cancerous sores the next year. He could not have predicted that his mind would start to turn on itself within months.

Once all of the family had arrived, my mother led the service, and everyone took turns saying something about my uncle. I read a poem about him that I had written in college. For once, I wasn't nervous about reading. The words came out clear and even, echoing off the white walls of the room and then returning back into the roof of my mouth:

Birdman, Springfield Hospital

The sea gulls shift their wings,
cocked eyes pulp-tight,
and try to glide between
the thick folds of wind as
they sight the bread
and tunnel in, plucking the soft
dough from his broken fingers.

They smell his arrival every late
afternoon, when the burnt sun

*is hidden behind the Solomon House,
when the other patients stagger
on the porch, some laughing,
some mute, some frightened
at the sudden spread of gray wings.*

*He ignores the faces on the porch,
their dry eyes, chattering teeth,
stopped throats, and clamps down
the marble steps to the open gazebo
where he sets the plastic bag down
and ceremoniously begins
to break the bread.*

*The birds circle and swoop,
an enormous rice paper origami,
smelling the crusts, sensing the torn
bites falling beneath his hand.
A man on the porch becomes anxious,
sputtering from behind his nervous beard,
he lifts his gray sleeves in flight.*

*They stare from behind the white
banisters, an assembly of dull points.
They watch the muscled dives,
lead wings dripping like storms,
the birds rising together
and then falling, curved and powerful,
calling out to their mark.*

*The birds hover high above the gazebo
as he picks up the empty bag
and heads back inside.
The patients move out of his way,
their heads down, silent,
their eyes as dark as hooded falcons
just returning from a hunt.*

Everyone was quiet after I finished reading. I heard my mother swallow and my father rub the tip of his shoe across the floor. My sister was staring at the ceiling. I looked down at my stomach and saw the baby kick. Suddenly, it all seemed ridiculous. My uncle wouldn't have cared about our tribute or the baby I was about to deliver the next morning. He would have been focused on the window, on the sea gulls that were circling outside, aimlessly, still hoping for a scrap of food.

~

That night I was aware of every dusty corner and every pair of underwear that I decided to leave at home as I double checked my bag and went down my list *one more time*. I wasn't just packing for a trip; I was packing for a new life.

To distract ourselves, we went out to dinner at *The Manor Tavern*, a cozy restaurant in the country. I looked around the room at the other diners who were all over sixty years old. There was an extremely wrinkled woman with just a puff of white hair and a walker parked next to her seat. She had to be close to one hundred years old. I kept glancing at her, wondering if she was once in my same position. Perhaps, over eighty years before, she had waited for her first child to make his painful entrance. Did she still remember the night her water had broken, her fear of dying suddenly present in the wet trickle running down her thigh?

My husband announced to the table next to ours that we were having a baby the next day. They congratulated us and I smiled, trying to adjust my butt to a more comfortable position on the chair.

I ordered soft crab sautéed over pasta. When it arrived, I bit the legs off one by one and felt the fresh crunch between my teeth. It was a small crab, caught right before molting, just the right time to be sautéed in a light dredge of flour and butter, and placed softly over a swirl of angel hair pasta with slices of thin carrot and zucchini. My husband ordered his usual: steak and a Miller Lite. We didn't stay long, but it did help to keep me distracted for an hour.

When we arrived back at our house my sister called to tell me her house manager was in the hospital, and that she had been elected to fill in as the manager of her halfway house for the next six weeks. She would be in charge of keeping track of all of the other women, making sure that each one had her meal assignment and taking privileges away from anyone who was not home by eleven p.m. She was nervous about the responsibility, she said, to hold the keys to so many lives other than her own. Nevertheless, she was also proud to be moving into step two this month. She had finally accepted step one: *We admitted that we were powerless over our addiction, that our lives had become unmanageable.* She explained how it was so much harder than it sounded, to admit your lack of control, to expose your own weaknesses.

She rushed off the phone because another housemate had to check in with her parole officer. She wished me a quick "Good luck tomorrow," and I heard the bland horn of the dial tone in my ear.

I picked up *Moby Dick*. I was still only halfway through the book, up to the chapter entitled, "The Funeral," which described the discarding of a sperm whale's carcass after it had been skinned and butchered. It was like all funerals, a mourning of loss and a celebration of renewal. The whalers bid farewell to the creature as the sharks and birds devoured their new feast. There were pages and weeks to go before the great white whale would surface again and blow his magnificent spout. I bookmarked my spot and made a mental note to remember to put the book in my suitcase in the morning, with the rest of my necessities for giving birth.

My husband's snoring woke me at midnight. I continued to wake up every hour after that. At 5 a.m., I finally gave up on sleep, climbed out of the bed and started my morning ritual. Every activity was in slow motion: my shower, brushing my teeth, rechecking the suitcase, feeding the dogs. I watched my hands doing the motions, disconnected from their movements. We finally left for the hospital around 7:30 a.m.. The last thing I did was to put the recycling out a day early, since we wouldn't be home the next night.

~

I walked up to the desk and waited for the admitting nurse to turn to me and smile, to declare that she knew it was the day for my child to be born, and that she was thrilled I had chosen her as the first memory of my hospital experience. Instead, she turned with a stiff face.

"Can I help you?"

"I'm here to have my baby," I stuttered. "9:30."

"Just a minute," she managed to return as she pulled out a stack of paperwork the size of a mortgage settlement. She fished through the papers for over two minutes. I looked around the empty lobby and tried to comprehend that I was there to give birth. It still didn't seem real. The stiff upholstered couches were reminders that it had to be a dream. The end tables were only short shadows, ghosts of past families waiting for good news, armed with balloons, flowers and teddy bears.

Finally, the admitting nurse found my sheet and ripped the printer edging off the sides. The rips were loud and rough.

"Sign here."

I barely glanced at the information as I scribbled my name and checked the square that stated I did not have a living will.

"You both need one of these," she said, as she held up two plastic I.D. bracelets. I tried not to shake as her cold hand slipped the bracelet around my wrist and pressed the extra plastic notch down to keep it attached. After my husband's bracelet was on, she directed us to the waiting room behind the double doors. I noticed the carpet looked brighter, like it had been cleaned since I had last waited there, ten months before.

"Maybe we should have brought the suitcase in," I said, trying to find a comfortable spot for my hands along the blue arm rests of my chair.

"I'll get it later," my husband replied, crossing his ankles and then uncrossing them.

"Oh no!" I stopped.

"What's wrong?" my husband turned in his seat.

"I forgot to bring *Moby Dick*! It's next to the bed. I wanted to finish it before I came home from the hospital!" I felt the tears starting.

"It's. . ." he started to say as a nurse peeked around the corner of the room and interrupted.

"You can come this way." We stood up, and I looked back at my chair twice before walking forward, without my suitcase or my book, towards the next set of double doors and the operating room that waited somewhere on the other side.

~

My clothes were in the clear plastic bag. My hair was up in the ponytail holder I had almost forgotten to bring. Neither of us knew what to say, as any words felt artificial and awkward. I counted the thick brushstrokes of the familiar yellow wildflower print on the wall. I was about to be cut open, and a baby was about to be released from my body. I was not there yet, though. I was *almost* there.

My husband pulled on his scrubs. It didn't even look like him. For a moment, I wanted to scream that it must be someone else's husband, only pretending to be my husband. I wanted to explain that I was not even supposed to be there, that there was actually no baby. The ultrasound was a mix-up, and my weight gain was just too many Oreo cookies. I had day dreamed the entire last year. I would wake up soon, and open my eyes to a world that I remembered, with clear focus and vision, and schedules that passed like clockwork.

I started to think of my escape route out the side door and down the staircase when a mustached nurse came in, raised my wrist to look at my I.D. bracelet and began to wash her hands in the sink.

"I am going to shave you first," she declared, and then glared over at my husband, who was staring at his feet.

"Good, you're dressed," she nodded her approval at his promptness, and started to pull up my hospital gown. She removed two inches of hair with a large silver blade that reminded me of my grandfather's razor, resting with a dull shine next to his aftershave.

"The incision will be right here," she pointed, then drew an imaginary line across my pelvis.

"All done," she smirked, as she patted my ankle. "Now it's time for the catheter."

"The *what?*" I asked.

She didn't answer me, but I started to get the picture as she began to unroll a flesh colored tube that was about as wide as a garden hose.

"Relax," she said, as she shoved cotton balls inside my vaginal lips.

When the target was wide open, she went in for the kill. I dug my nails into my husband's hand and screamed.

"That was awful," I cried, as she wound up the tube of torture and fastened it to the side of the bed.

She chuckled as she continued her organization, pulling out tape, towels, and labeling bags and pieces of paper with my name and insurance information. I twisted my plastic I.D. bracelet around my wrist, trying to recover from the pain. I spun it around three more times for good luck, just like I used to do with my high school class ring.

~

Somewhere outside the room, down the sterile hall, through the second set of double doors, out in the waiting room, on one of the striped couches, my mother was waiting, pretending to be reading a *Fit and Healthy over Fifty* magazine.

She was remembering my birth, the long hours spent chipping paint flakes off the labor room window as the contractions slowly crept closer together.

She was alone, my father left to stare at the black and white television in the waiting room with the other expectant fathers. The room was off-white, the shade of aged bone, and she couldn't find anything to distract her from the pain. She kept thinking of the miscarriage, of the clot baby that had slipped out in the toilet. She wondered if the clot baby might actually be this baby. Maybe the baby had just not been ready to come down to earth the first time. Maybe the baby had just needed more time in the preexistence before it shed its gauzy memory veil and passed into this world. My mother didn't think that she would ever move beyond that moment. That is what her whole life had been leading up to: that moment, that second. She scraped off enough of the white flakes from the painted window to see two nurses walking across the courtyard of the hospital in their long white dresses and stiff hats. She couldn't understand how it was possible, how people could still be going about their days, walking, talking, and breathing. Her world was so small. Just herself, the window, and the child she had not yet met.

~

The nurse wheeled me into the cold chill of the surgery room. There were metal cabinets everywhere, cold gray cabinets that matched the masks covering everyone's faces. The anesthesiologist complained about *The Orioles* latest bad streak as he inserted my spinal. It only stung for a second, nothing like the blunt force of the catheter. The staff assembled around me as two of the nurses positioned me on the top of the table. They looked like curious aliens, their eyes the only characteristics distinguishing one person from the next. It took me a few seconds to register the doctor with the dark eyebrows was my own doctor, though he was not talking to me, he was talking to one of the nurses about his upcoming vacation. The nurse was laughing as she set a gray curtain veil up in front of my face.

Then there were only voices, all distant, all talking about things outside of the room, ordinary things like renovations and new food items at the cafeteria. My breath started to quicken, and I felt a small tug at my belly as someone straightened the surgery sheet. The bottom half of my body started to go numb. My husband was suddenly there at my head, camera in hand, and he snapped a profile of my face, sweaty with the oxygen tubes that had somehow made their way into my nose.

"They've already started cutting you," he said, looking over the curtain and snapping another shot. All I could feel was a light sensation rubbing across my belly. Then the weight on my upper body became more intense, like a cinder block was resting on my lungs. All I could see was the gray curtain sheet and the tiny fibers in the fabric that crisscrossed like a tight puzzle. My husband continued to snap pictures. I felt my cheeks becoming wet.

One of the nurses poked her masked face over the curtain and told me that I would be feeling a lot of pressure. I found a random red thread in the gray curtain and followed its path until it disappeared. I heard another one of the nurses make a joke about the new dry cleaning company. The room grew spottier and the weight shifted on my chest. The camera flashed. There was another tug.

"Almost," a voice I did not recognize announced on the other side of the curtain. And then, for a moment, there was pure silence: no talking, no voices, no language, and no movement. My breath was about to fill back into my lungs, my husband was just about to lose a tear, and the menacing silver operating tools were just out of sight, paused for a second in their duties.

~

I couldn't see him yet, as I was still behind the gray curtain wall, but I could hear him. He was screaming his first sound, a terrified response to the sharp sting of air against his raw lungs. It was the cry of a separate human being. It wasn't my voice. It wasn't my husband's voice. It was a voice I had never heard before.

I couldn't understand how the silence was now filled with sound, how before there was no one and now there was someone. I didn't know how the world had opened up enough space for another body. I only knew that he was suddenly there, and that the room shuttered with his high pitch. For the first time, seeing him didn't matter. I didn't need to see him to know everything would be all right. I would be able to hold him soon. *I would take care of him.* That was the first describable moment of his life, the first moment that he was finally real to me, and I closed my eyes to help remember the sound.

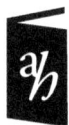

The future of publishing...today!

Apprentice House is the country's only campus-based, student-staffed book publishing company. Directed by professors and industry professionals, it is a nonprofit activity of the Communication Department at Loyola Univeristy Maryland.

Using state-of-the-art technology and an experiential learning model of education, Apprentice House publishes books in untraditional ways. This dual responsibility as publishers and educators creates an unprecedented collaborative environment among faculty and students, while teaching tomorrow's editors, designers, and marketers.

Outside of class, progress on book projects is carried forth by the AH Book Publishing Club, a co-curricular campus organization supported by Loyola University's Office of Student Activities.

Student Project Team for *Halfway: A Journal through Pregnancy*

Alyssa DeLisio, '10

Stephen Gallagher, '11

Alanna McGeary, '10

Amanda Merson, '10

To learn more about Apprentice House books or to obtain submission guidelines, please visit www.ApprenticeHouse.com.

Apprentice House
Communication Department
Loyola University Maryland
4501 N. Charles Street
Baltimore, MD 21210
Ph: 410-617-5265 • Fax: 410-617-2198
info@apprenticehouse.com

www.ingramcontent.com/pod-product-compliance
Lightning Source LLC
Chambersburg PA
CBHW071659090426
42738CB00009B/1589